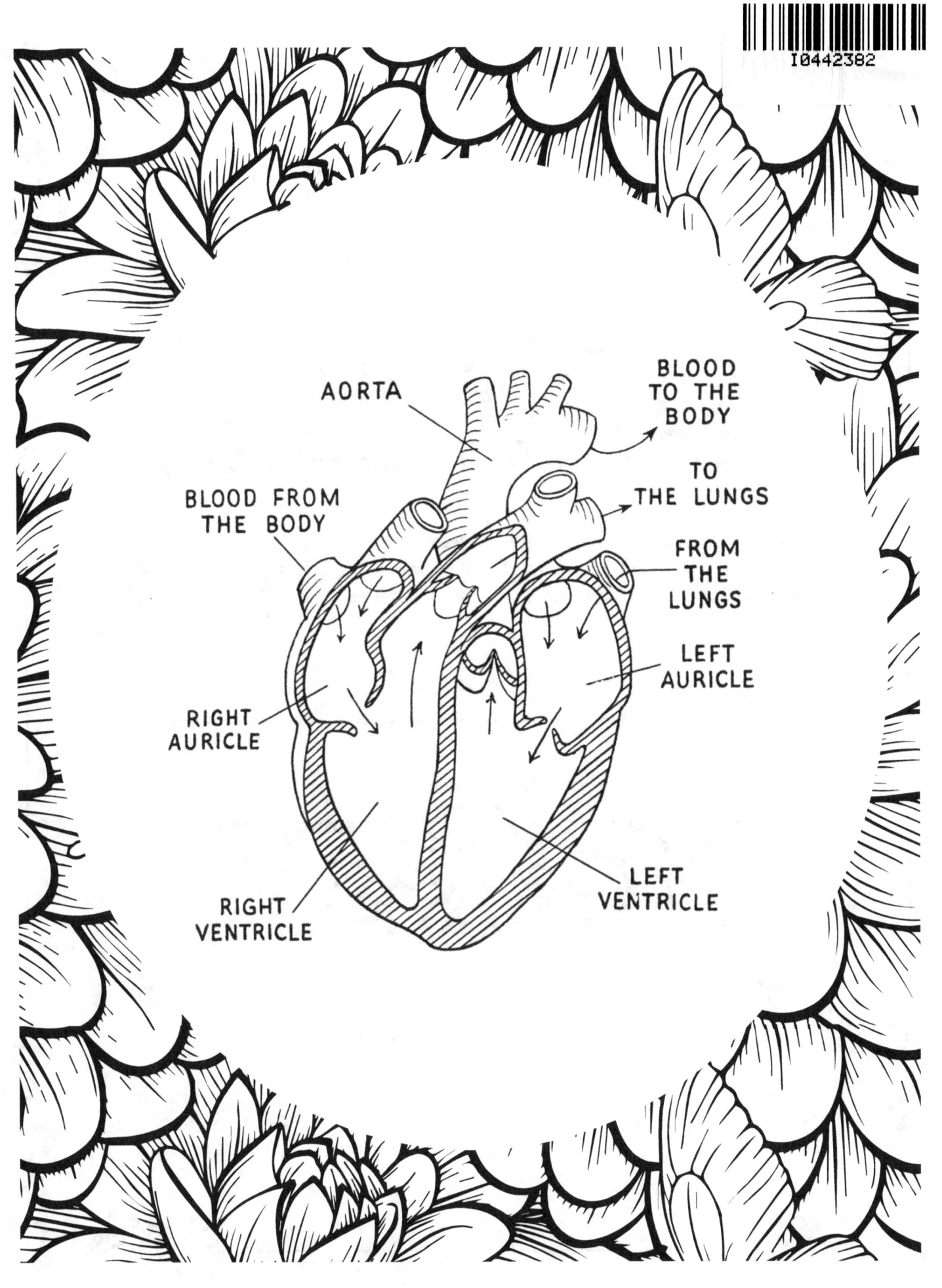

This Book Belongs To

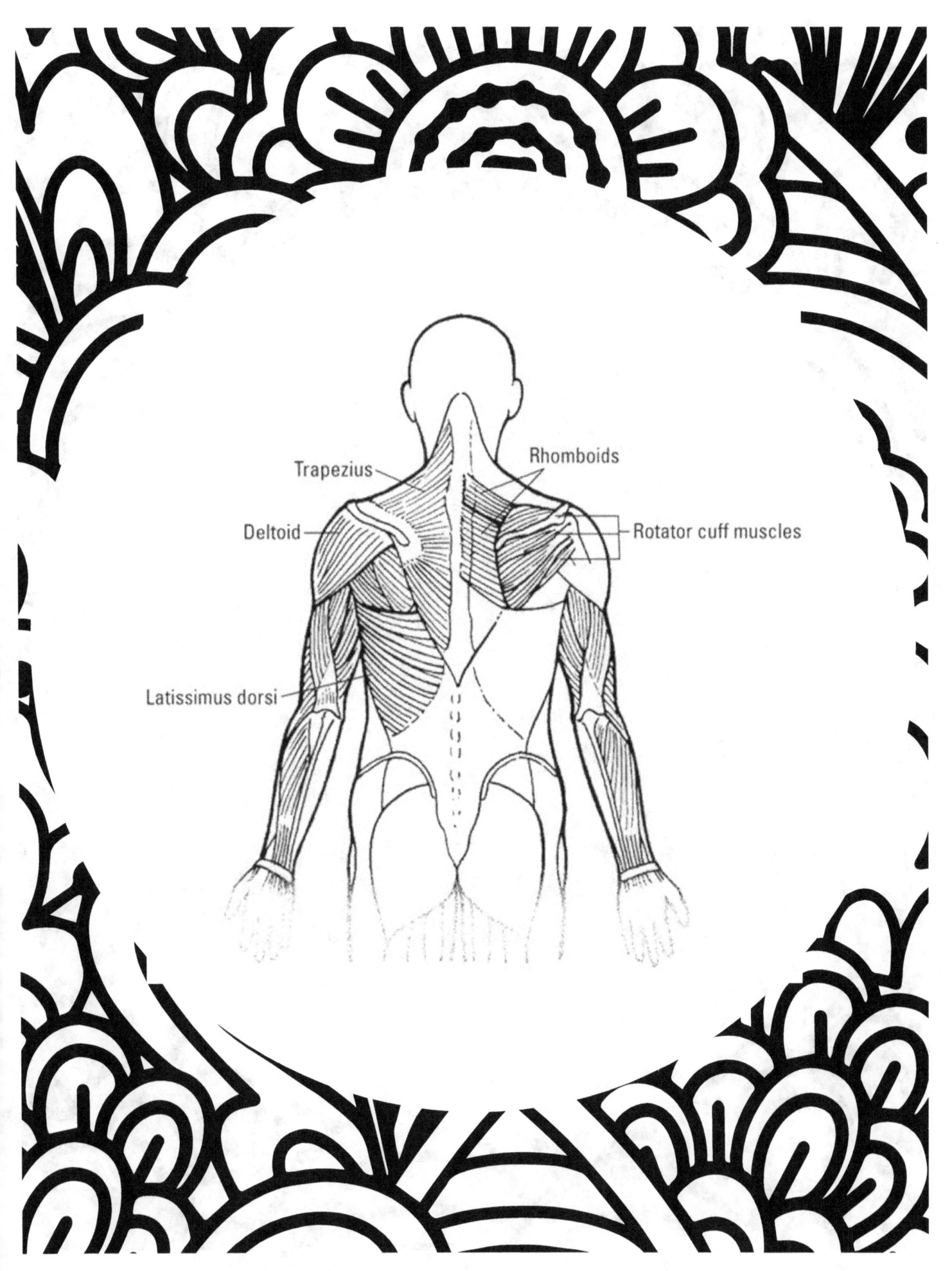

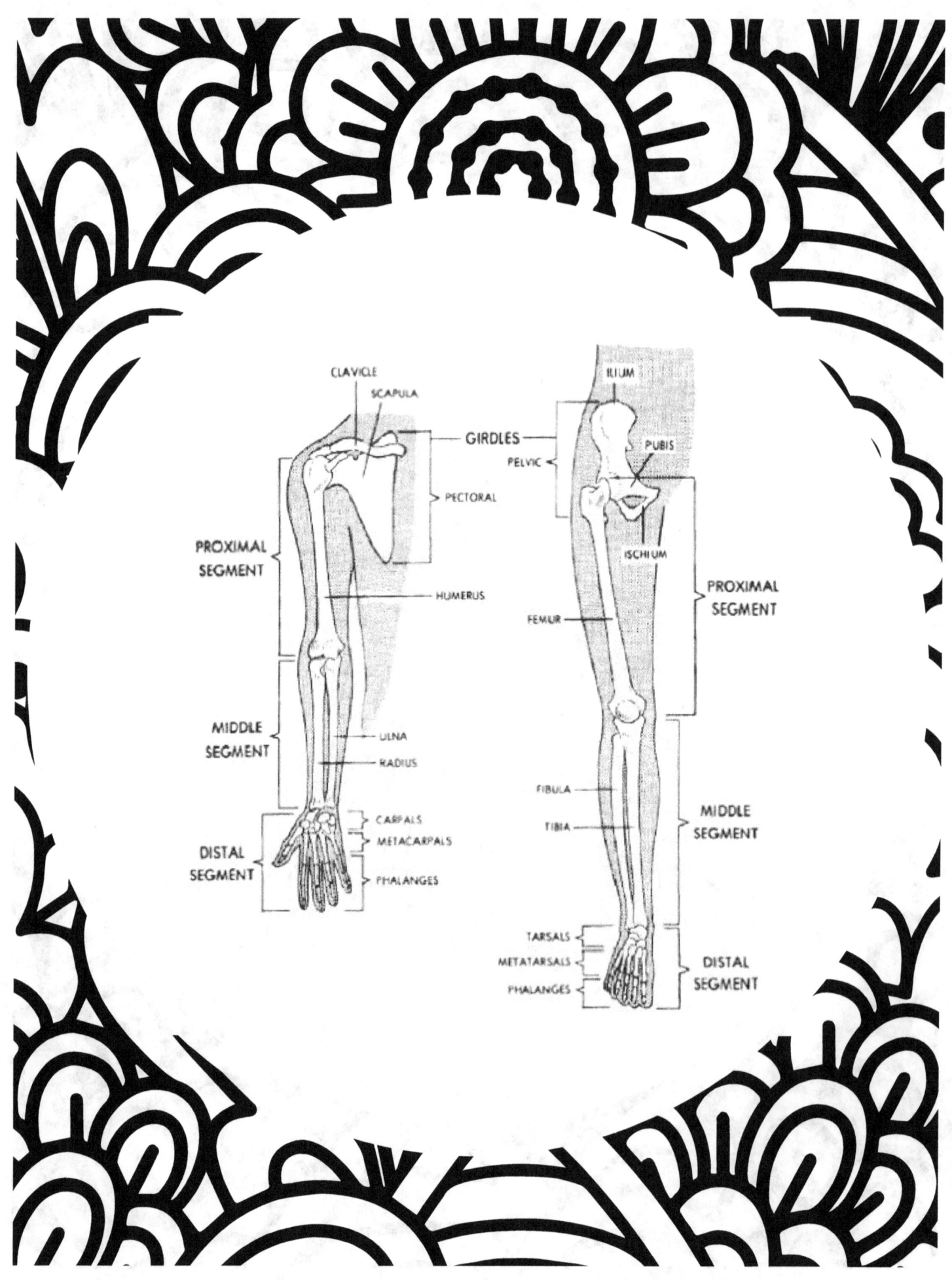

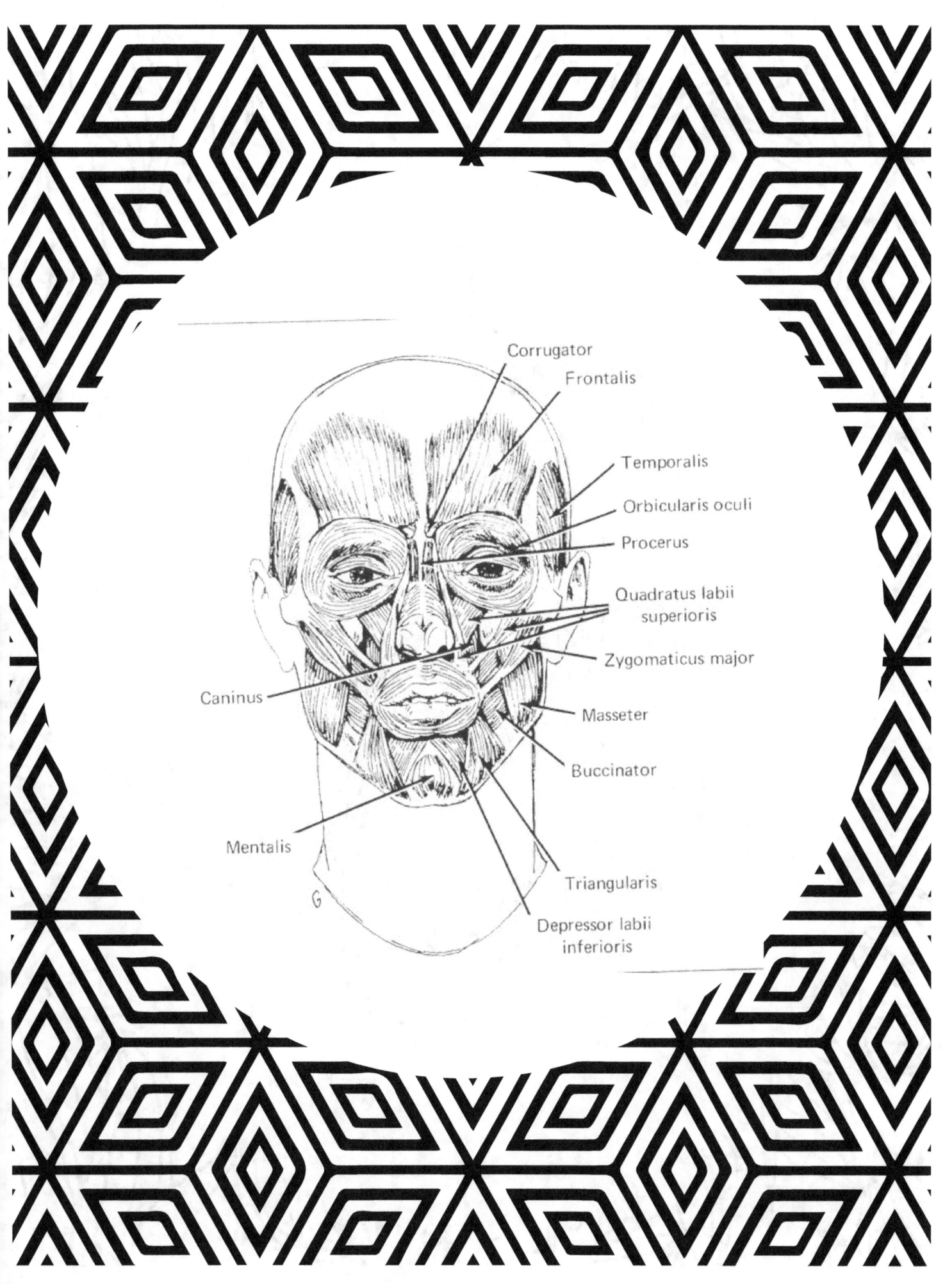

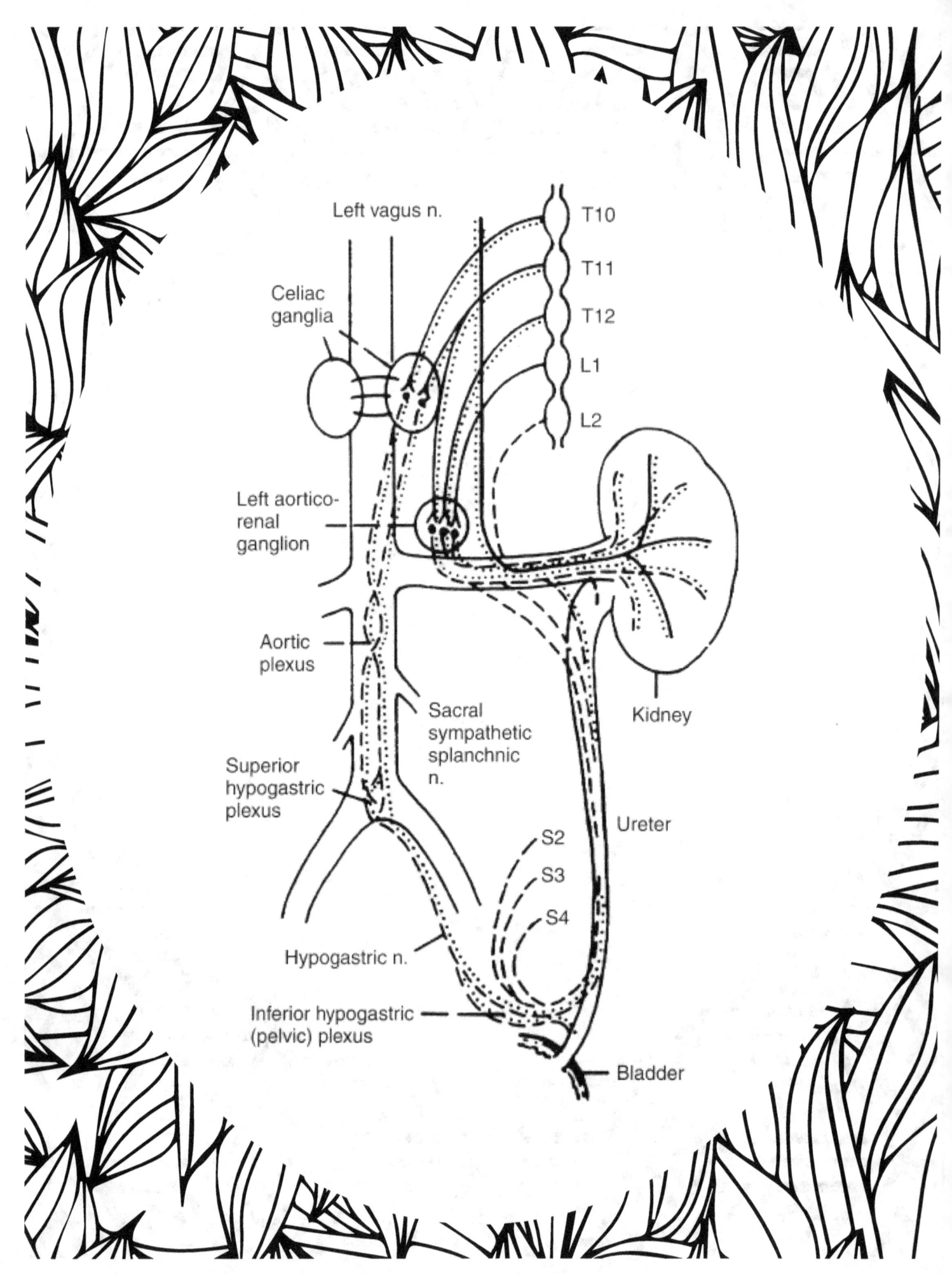

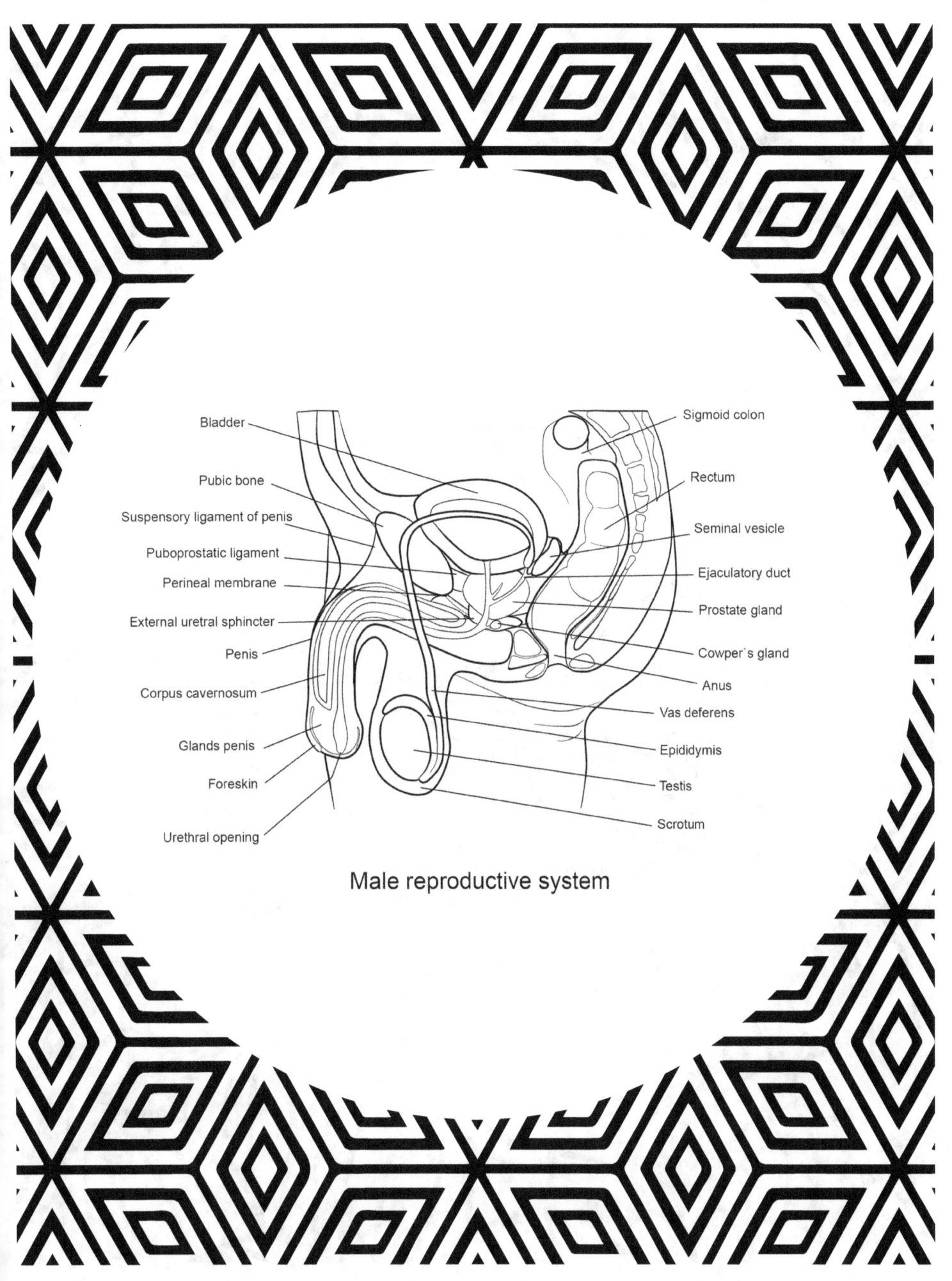

Male reproductive system

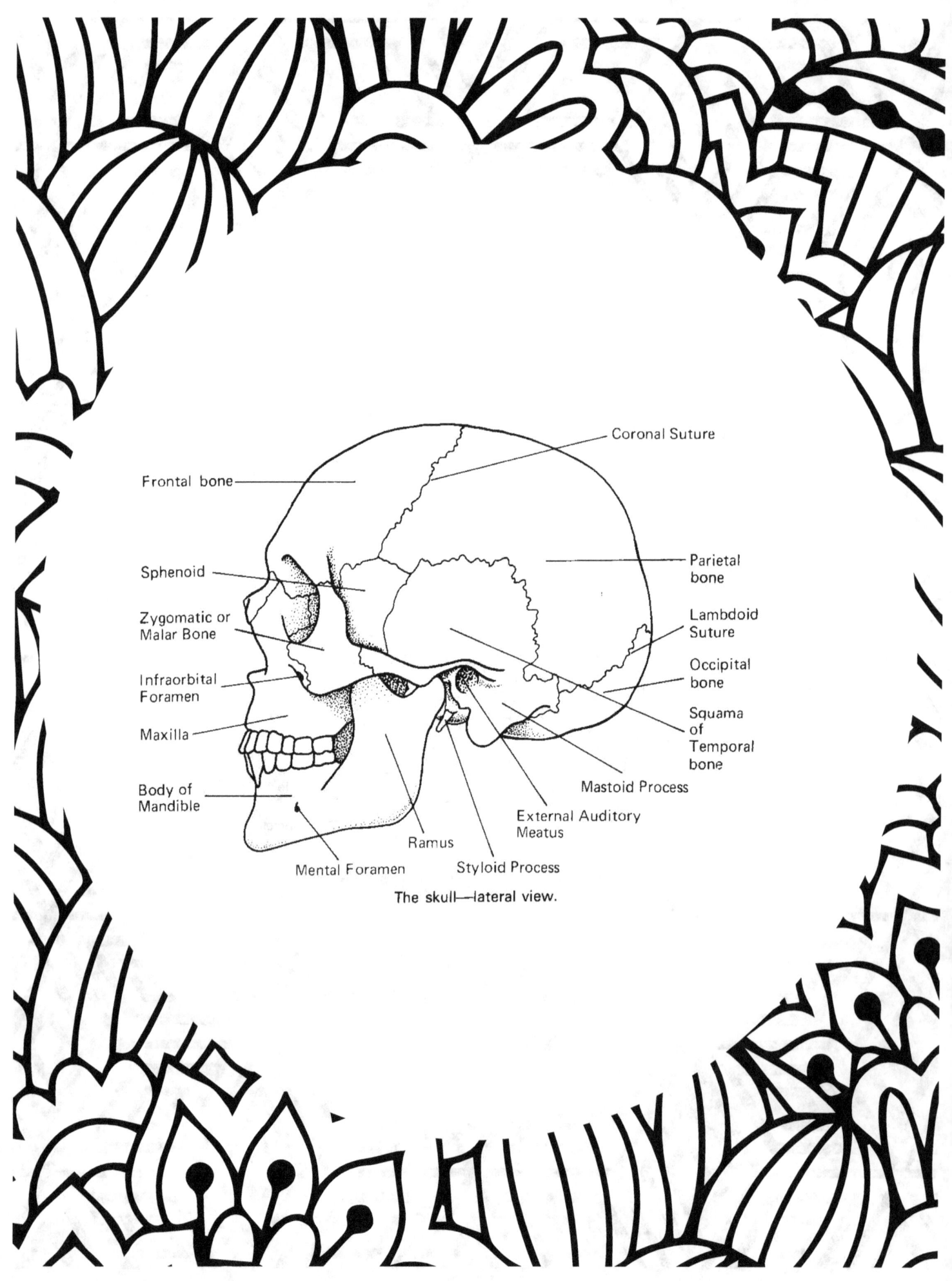

The skull—lateral view.

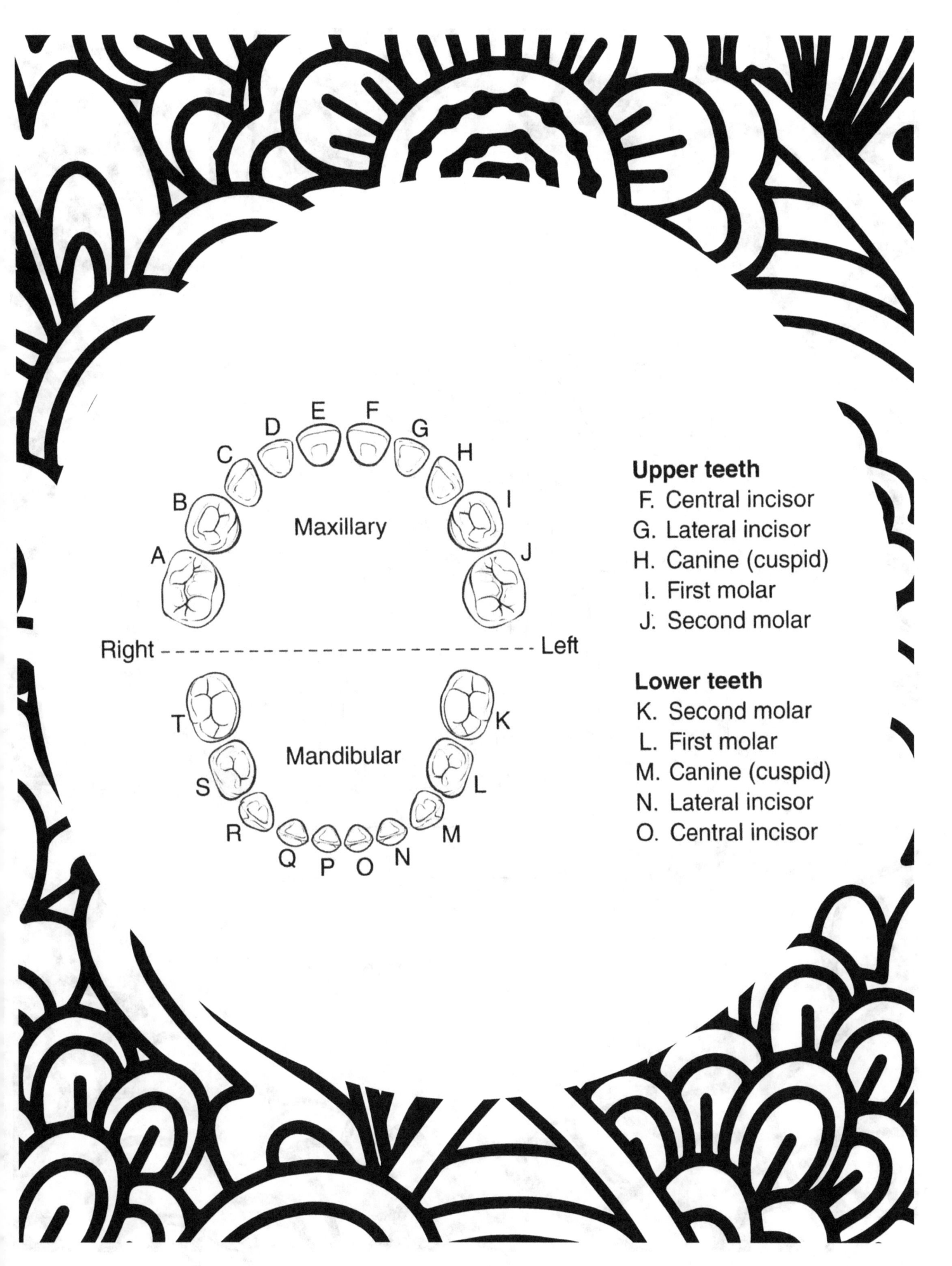

Upper teeth
 F. Central incisor
 G. Lateral incisor
 H. Canine (cuspid)
 I. First molar
 J. Second molar

Lower teeth
 K. Second molar
 L. First molar
 M. Canine (cuspid)
 N. Lateral incisor
 O. Central incisor

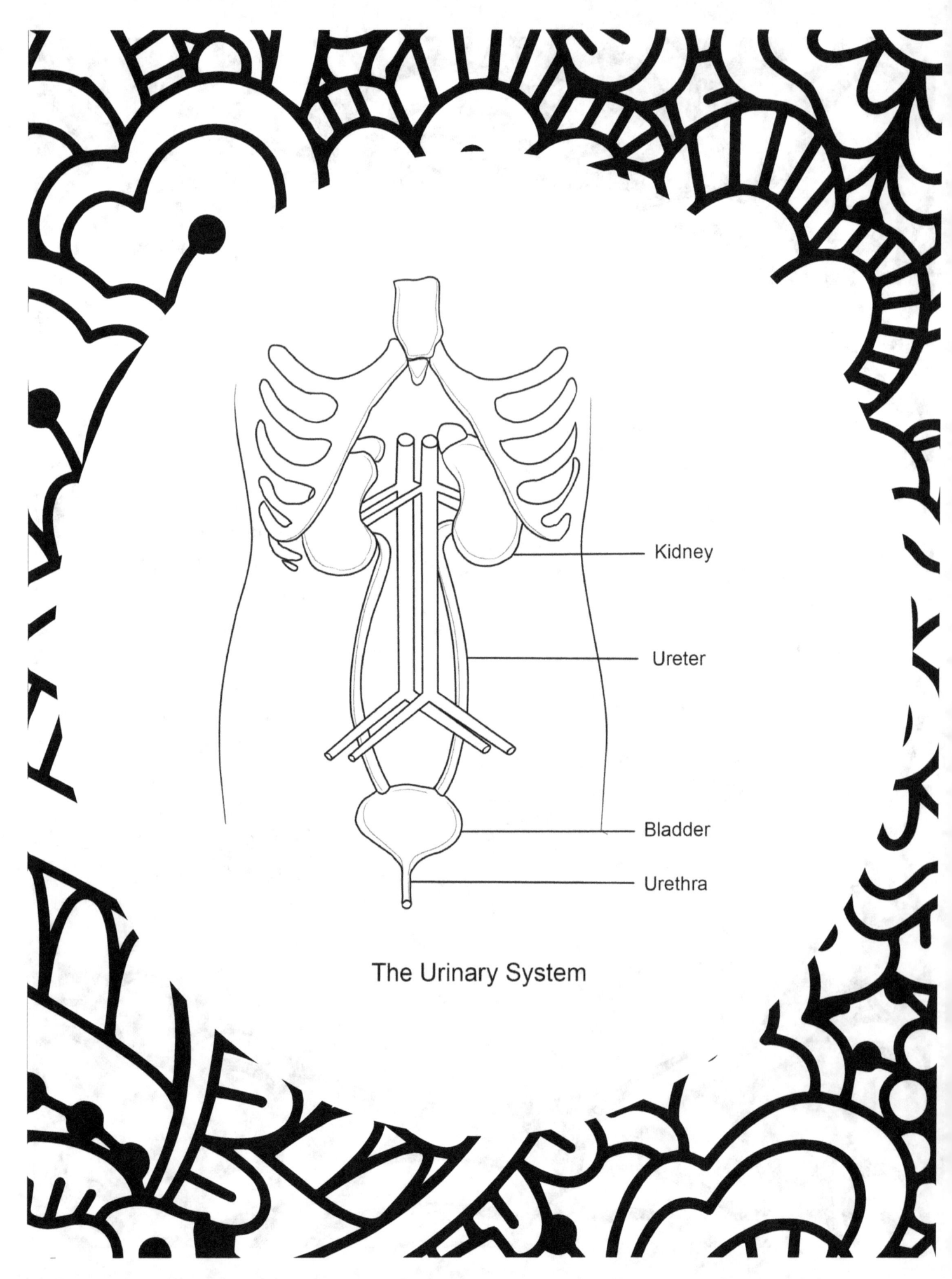

Kidney

Ureter

Bladder

Urethra

The Urinary System

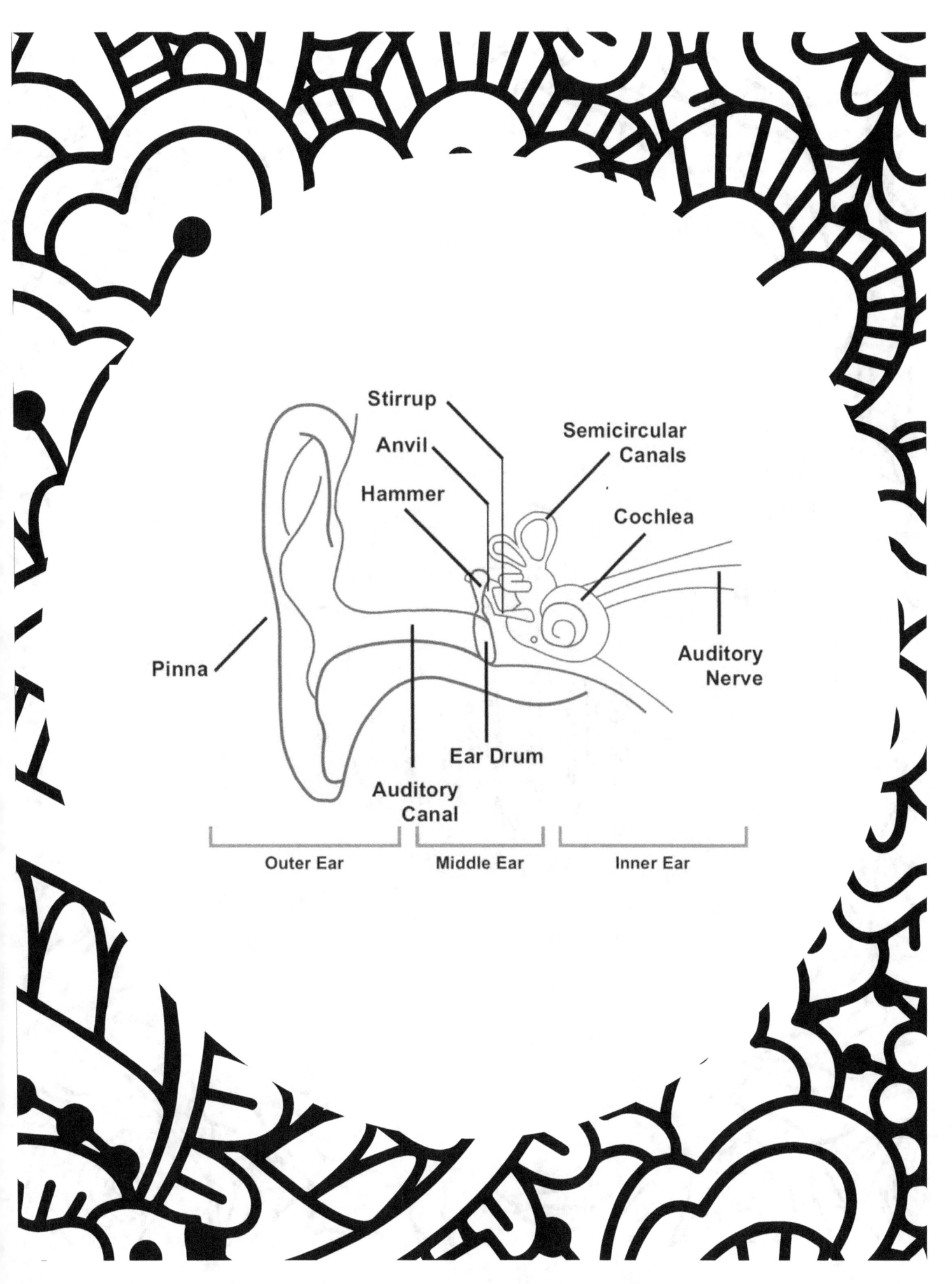

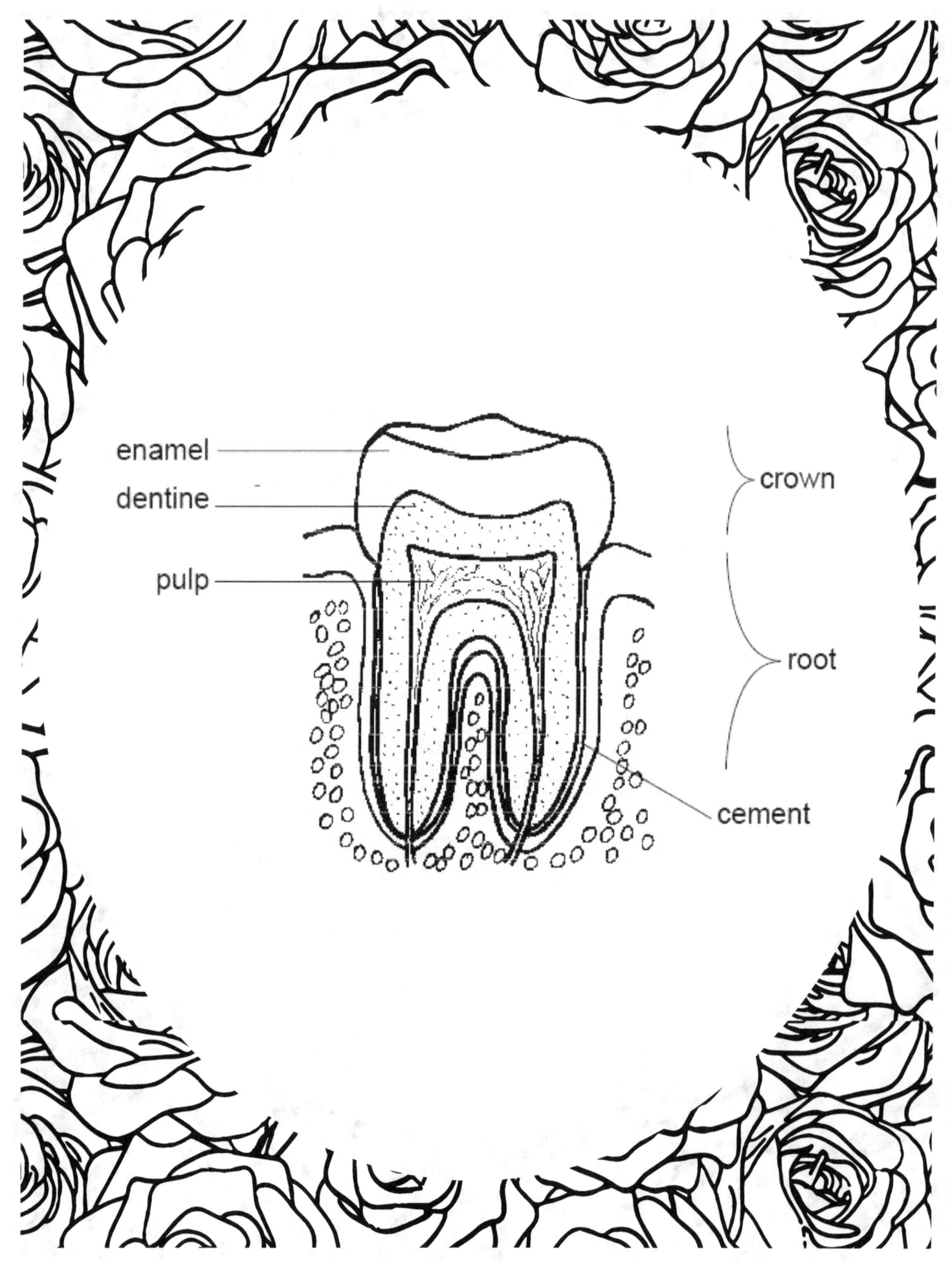

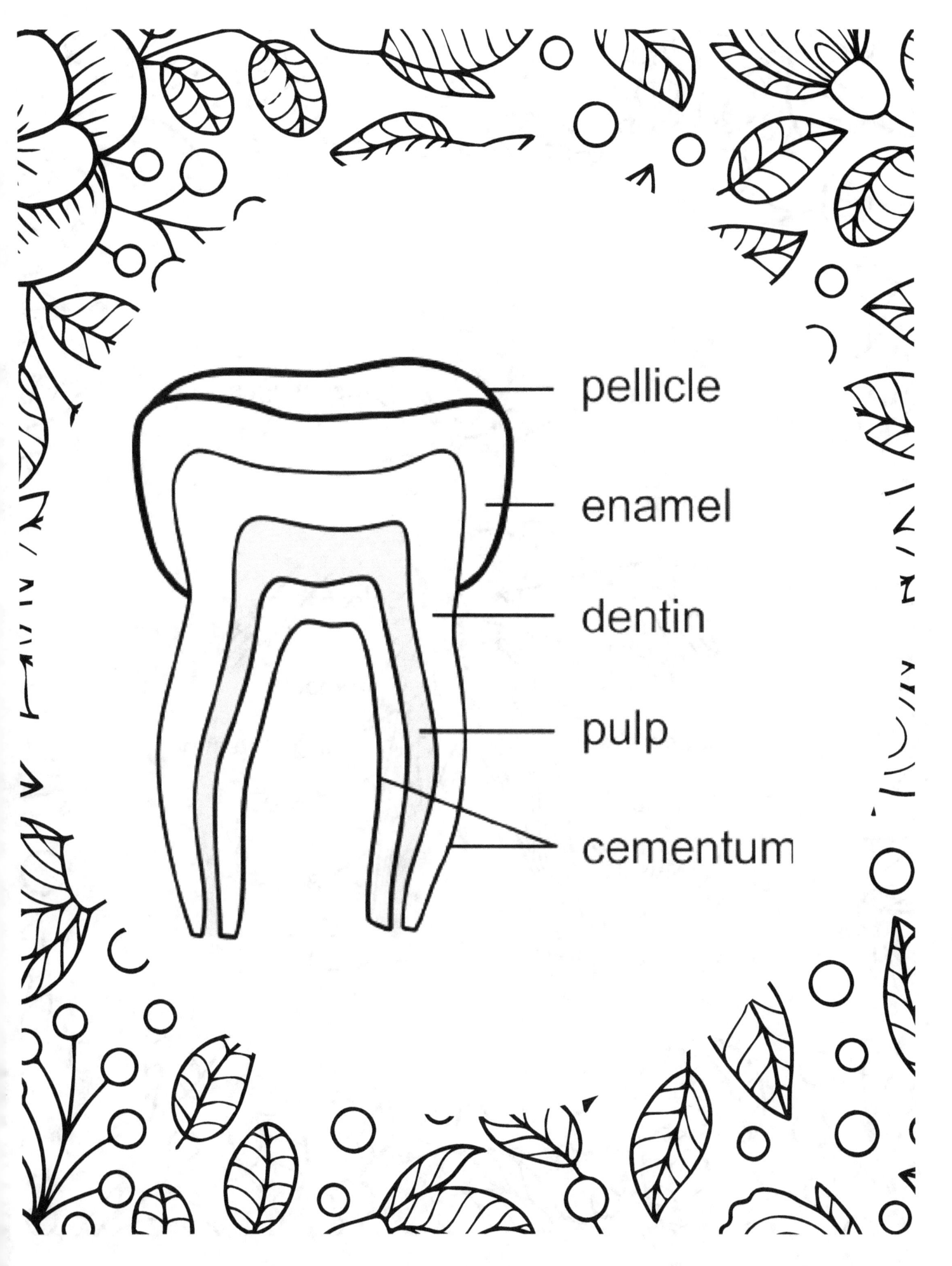

pellicle

enamel

dentin

pulp

cementum

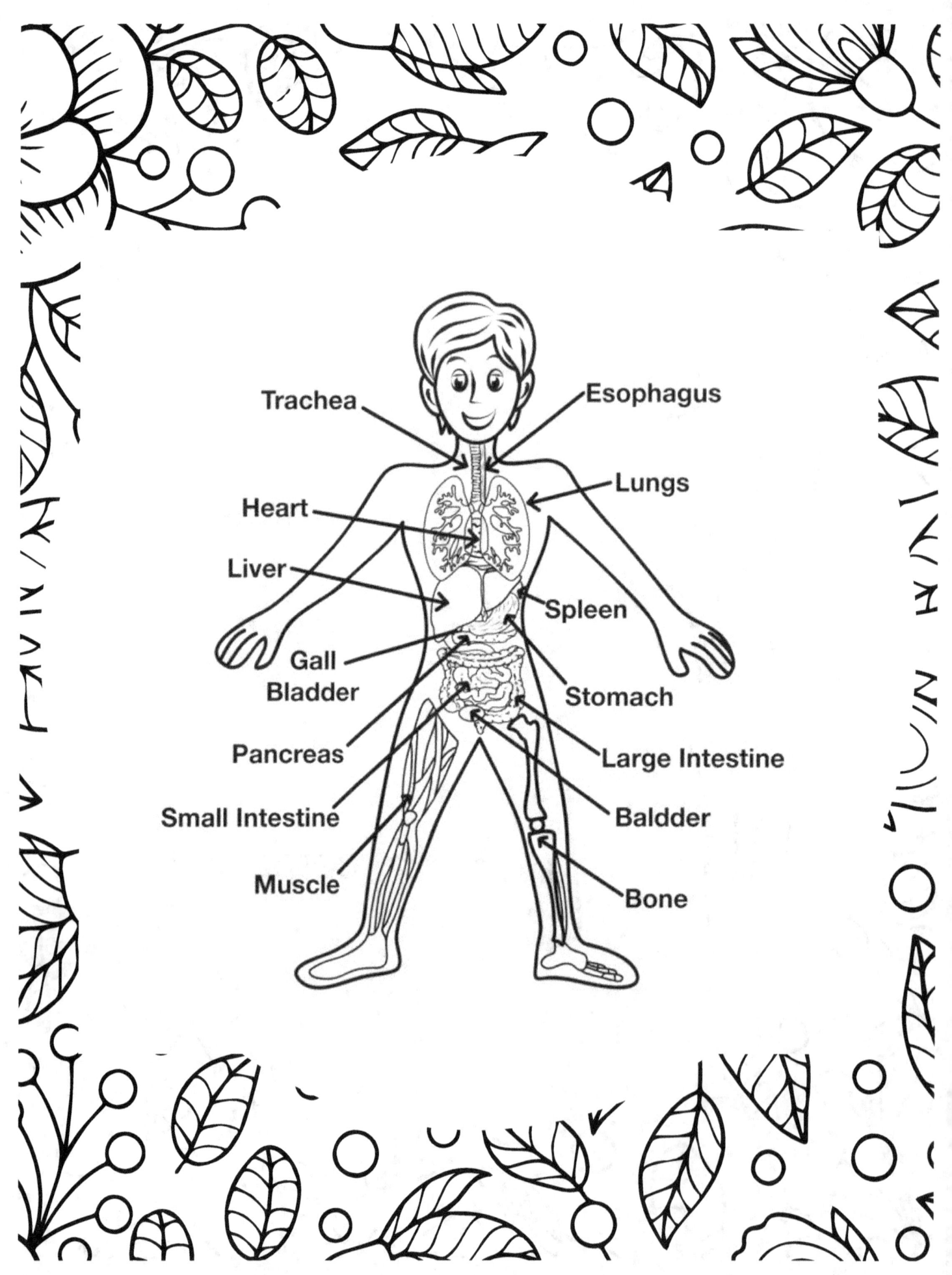

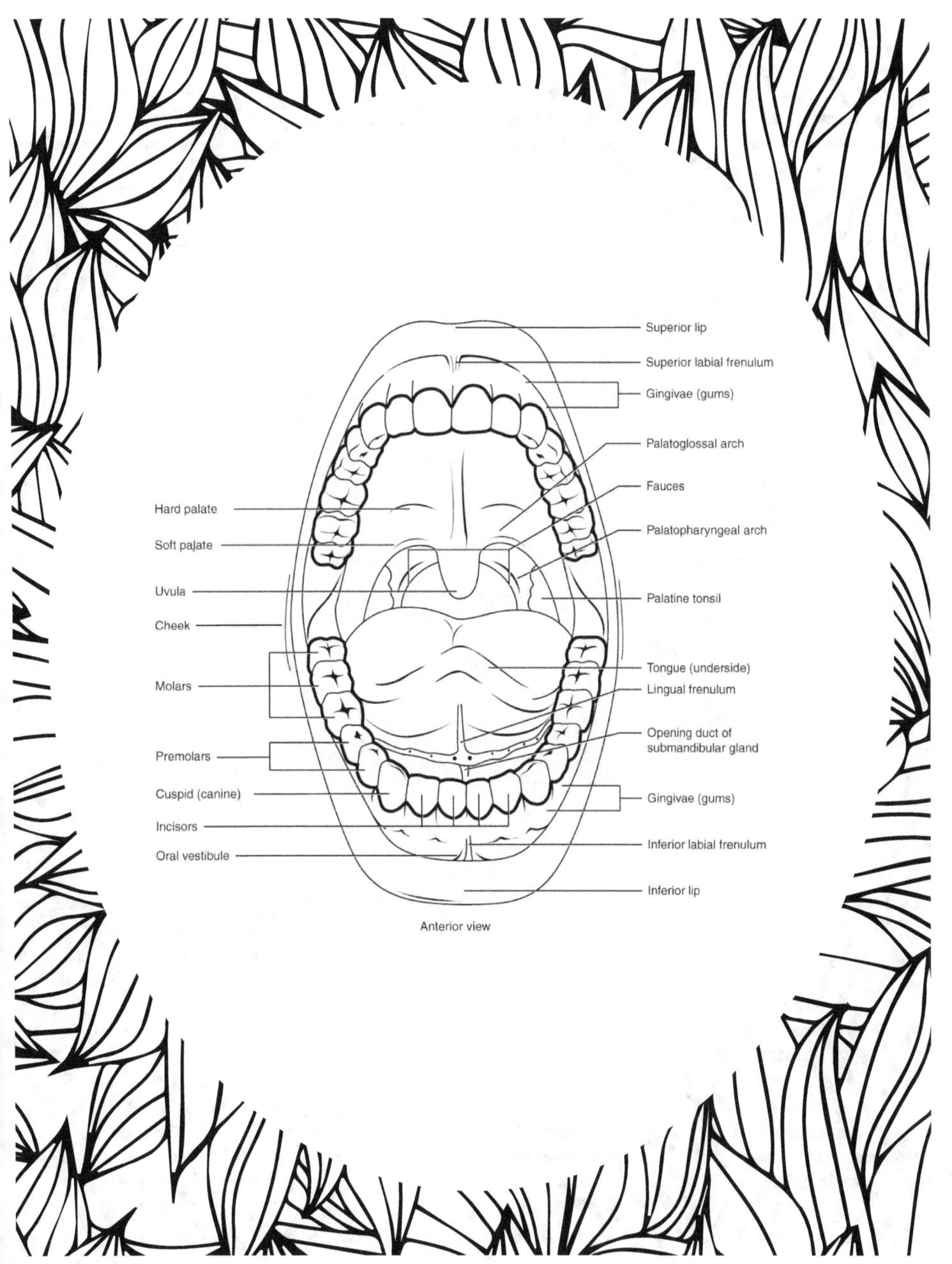

Superior lip

Superior labial frenulum

Gingivae (gums)

Palatoglossal arch

Fauces

Palatopharyngeal arch

Hard palate

Soft palate

Palatine tonsil

Uvula

Cheek

Molars

Tongue (underside)

Lingual frenulum

Opening duct of
submandibular gland

Premolars

Cuspid (canine)

Gingivae (gums)

Incisors

Inferior labial frenulum

Oral vestibule

Inferior lip

Anterior view

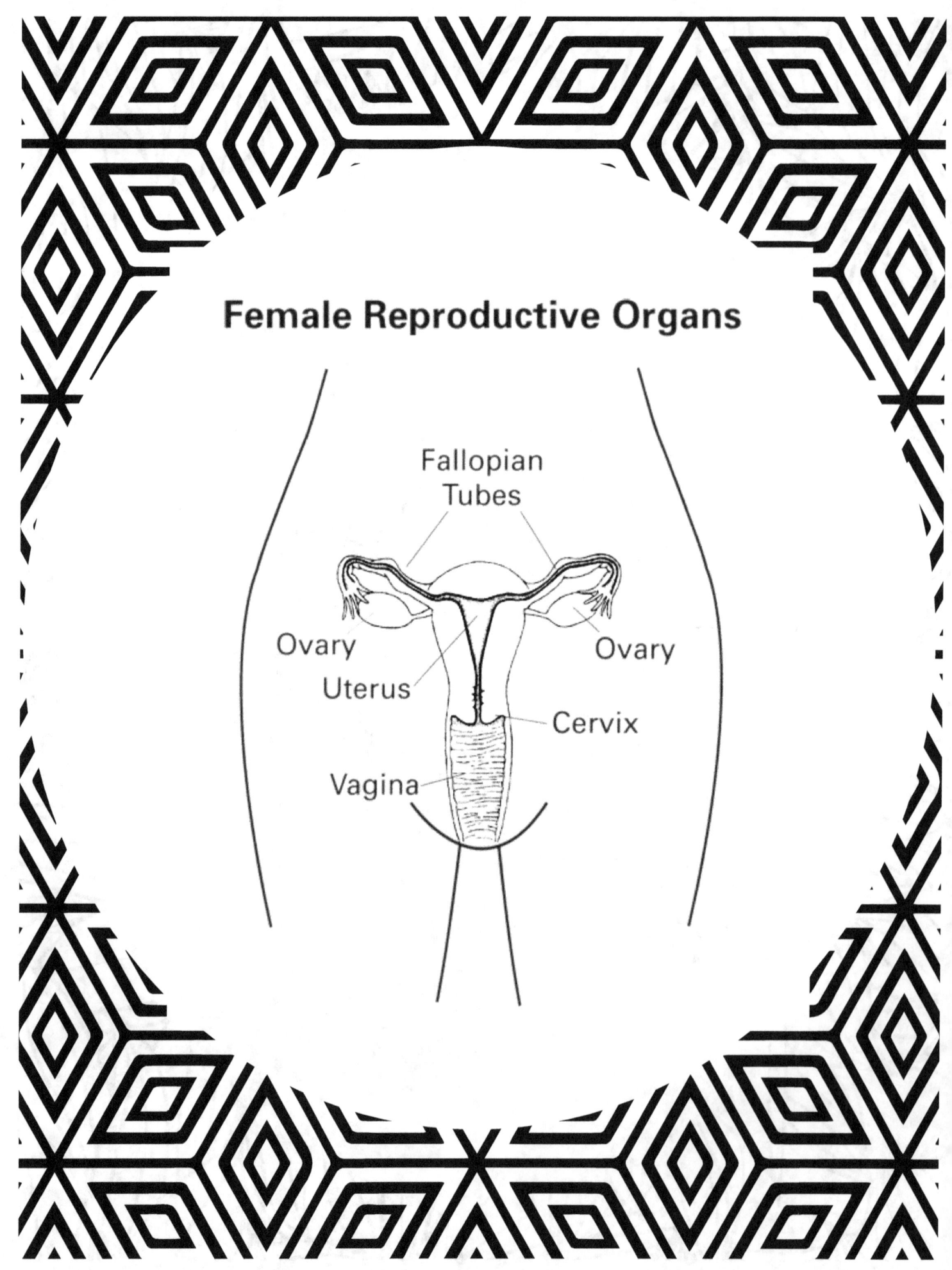

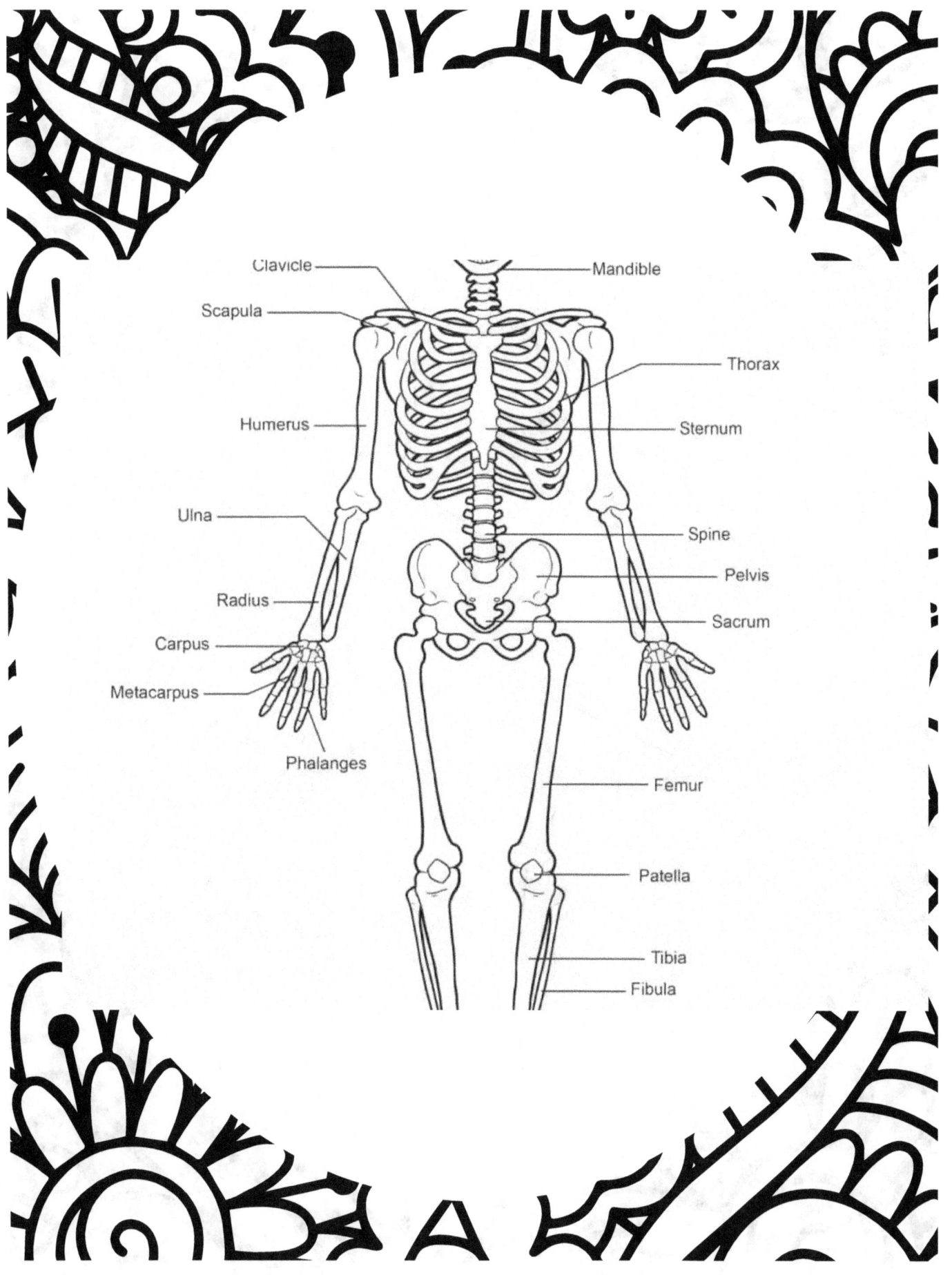

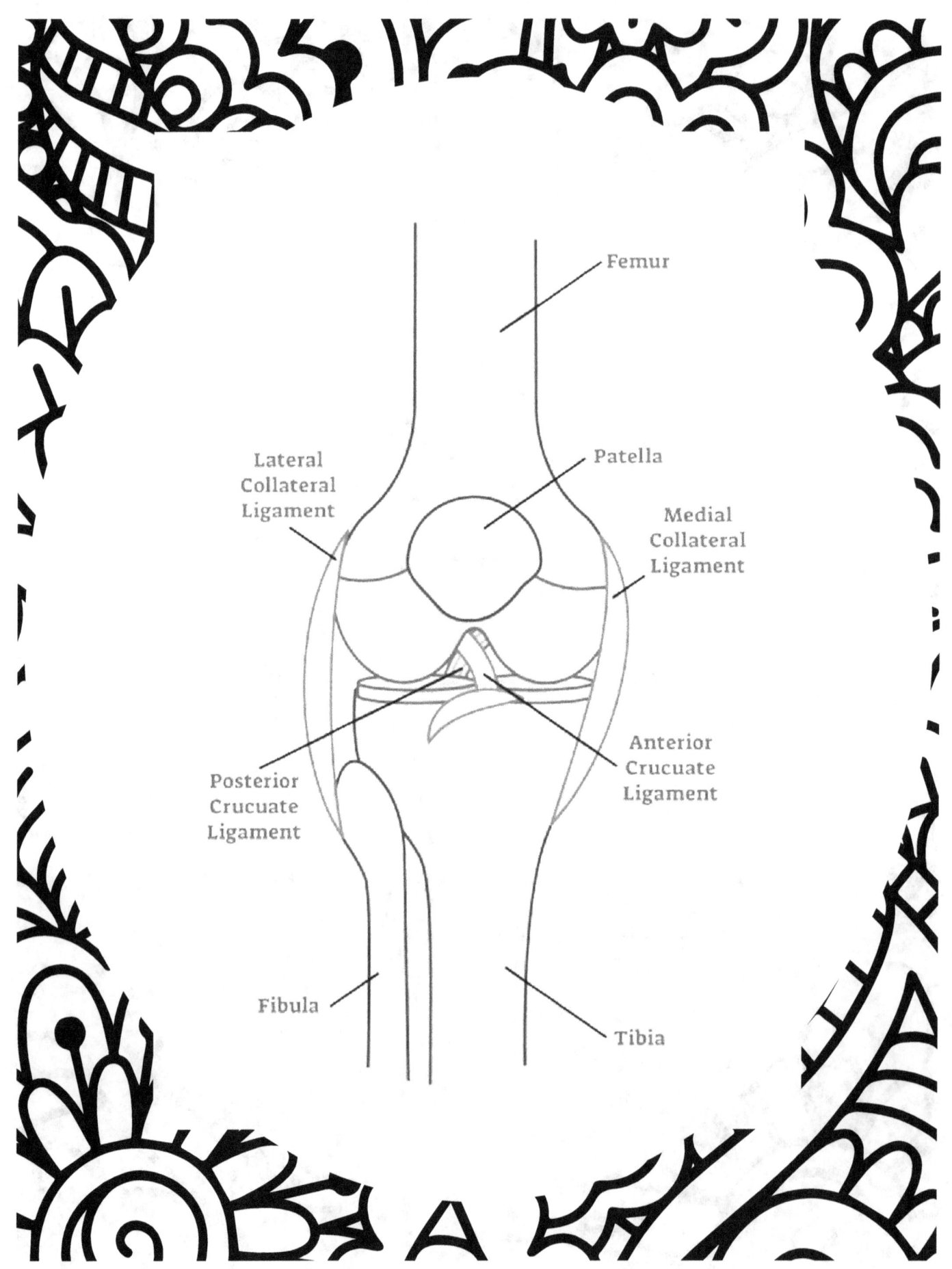

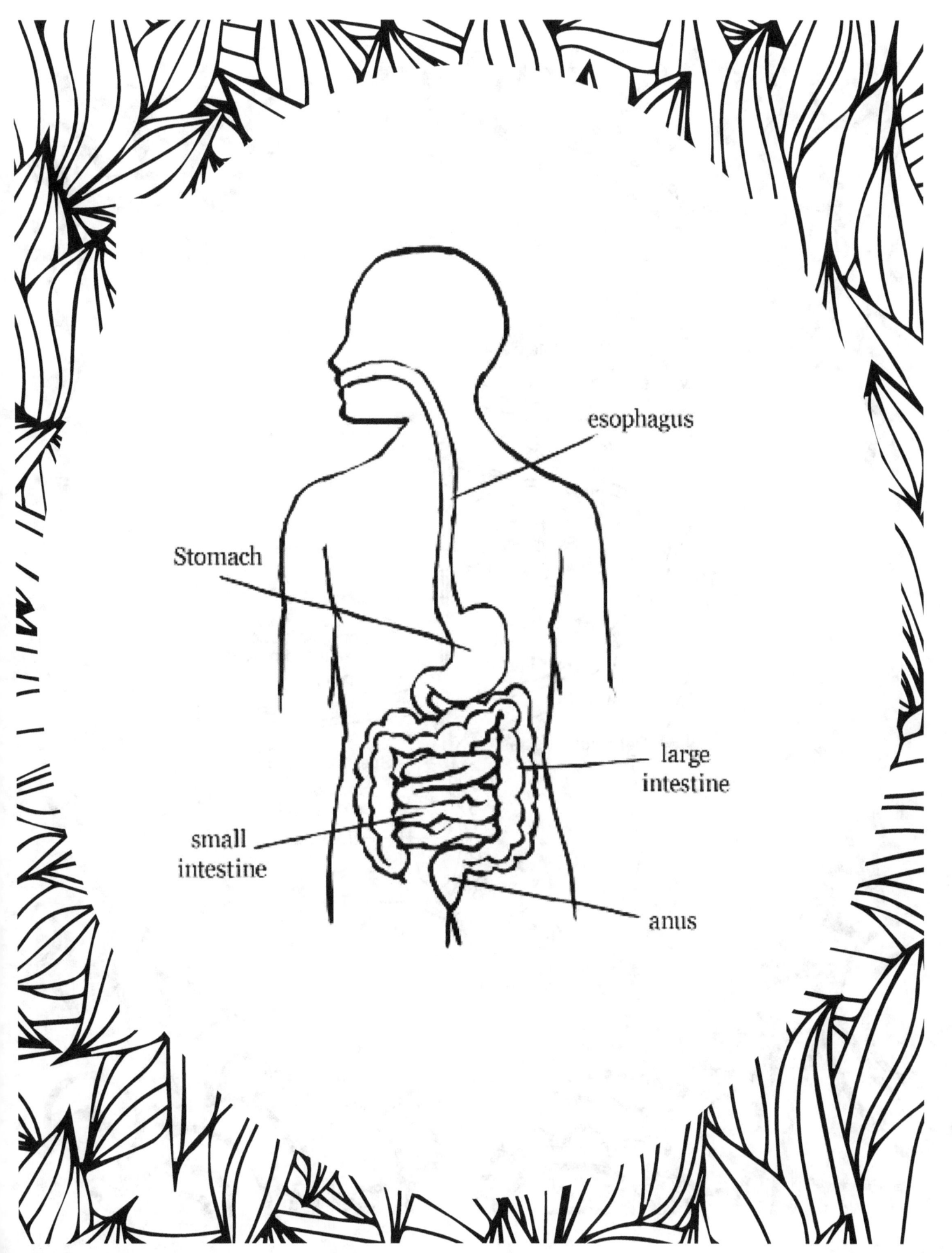

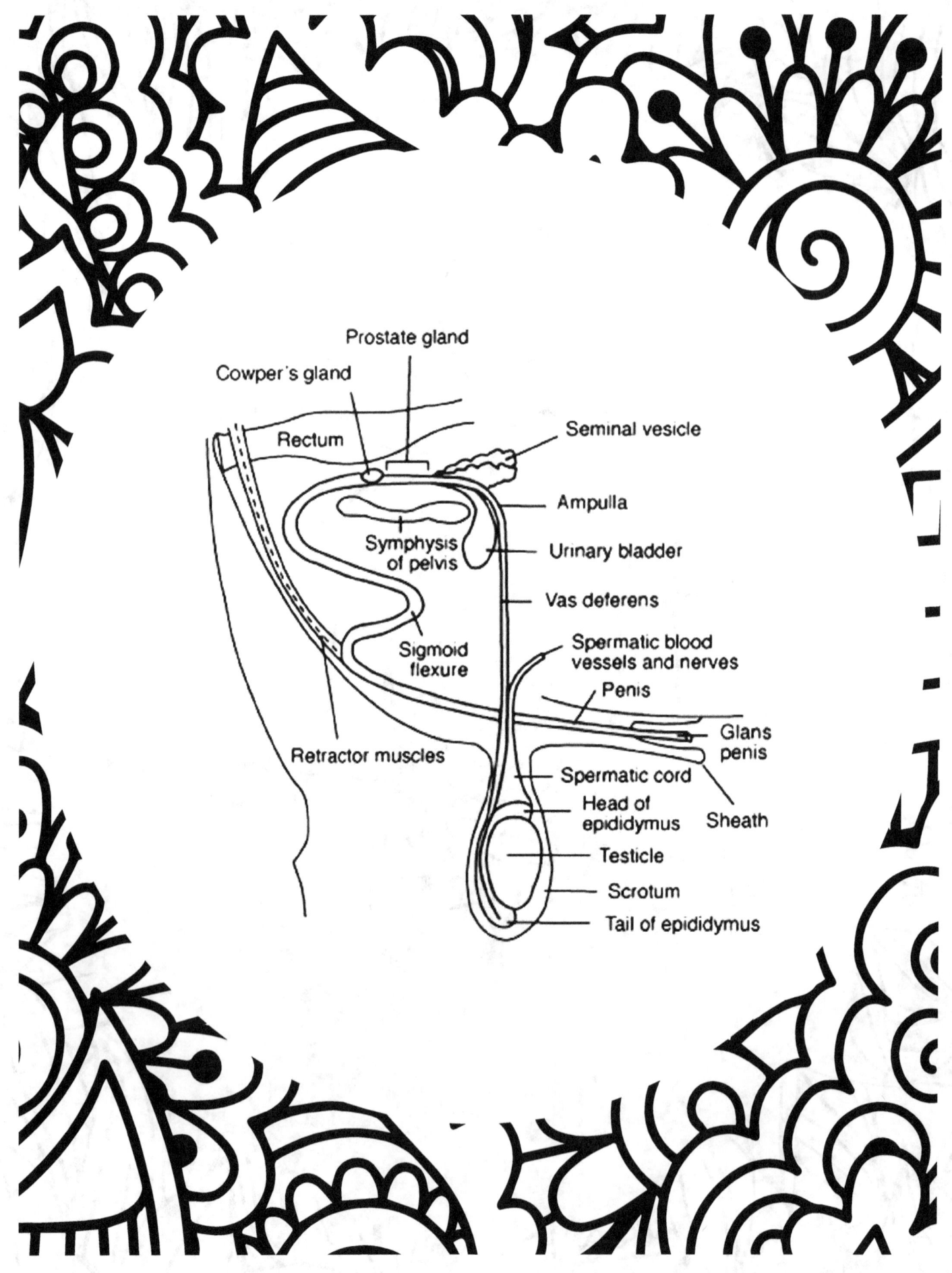

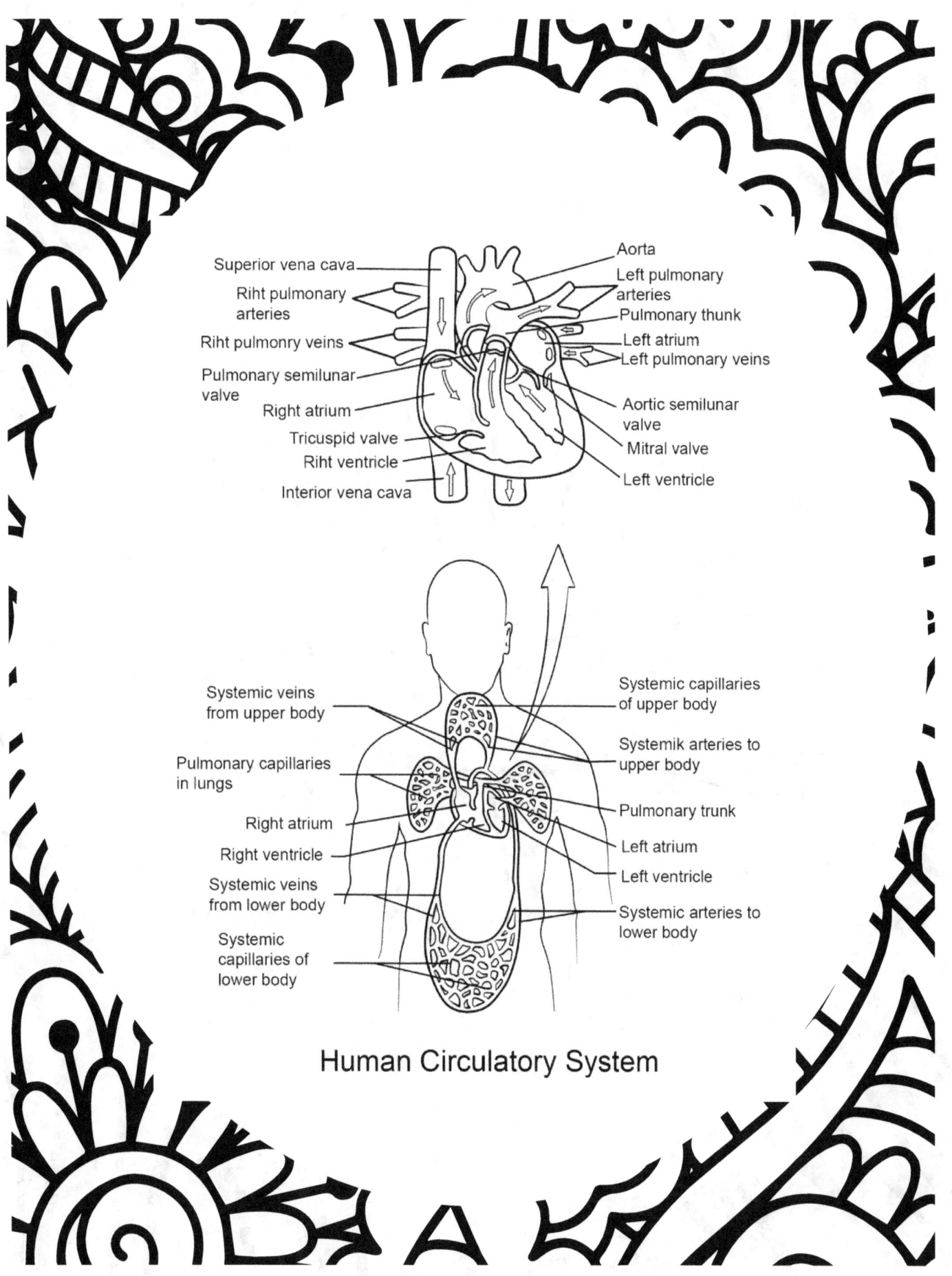

Human Circulatory System

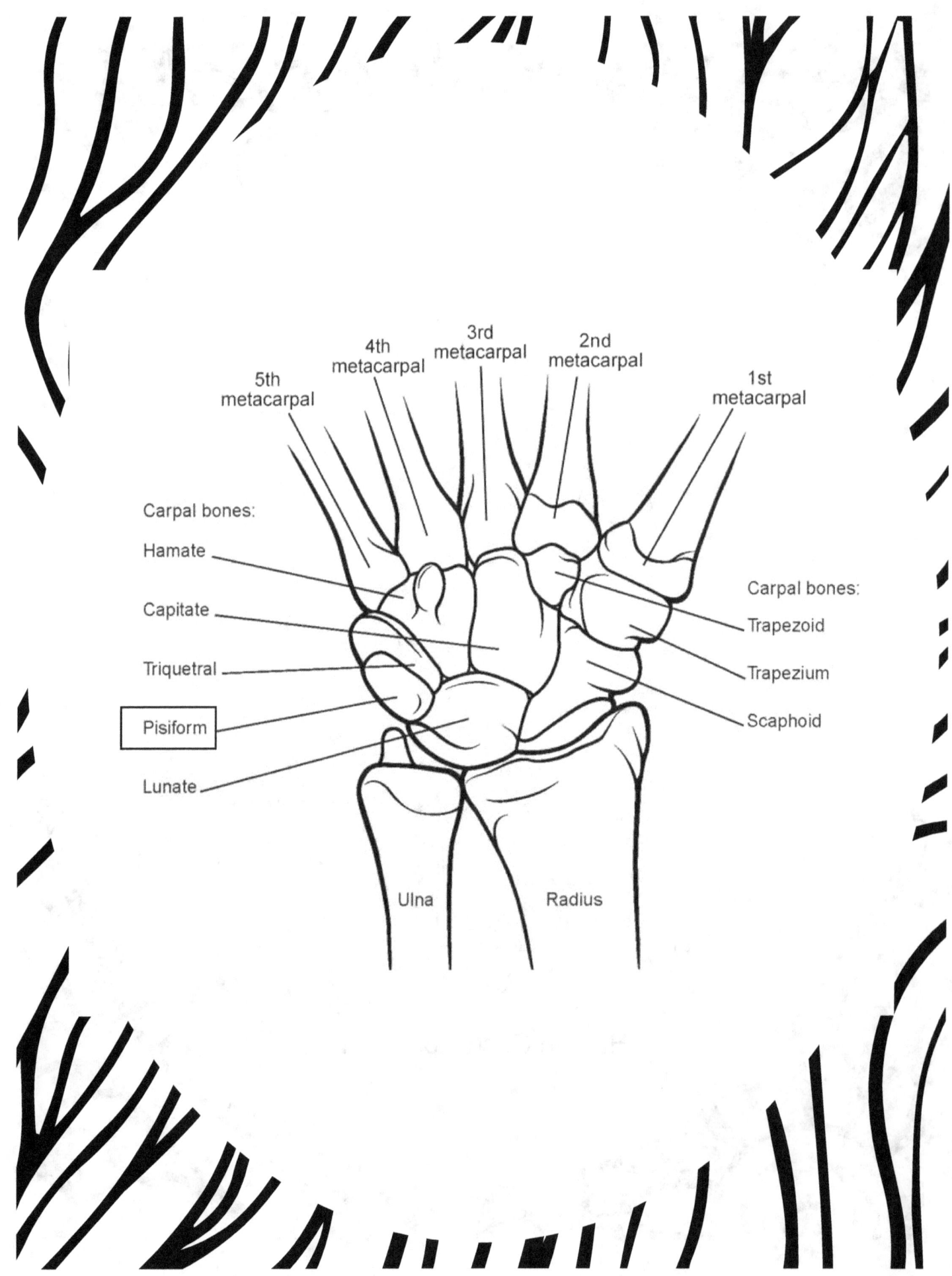

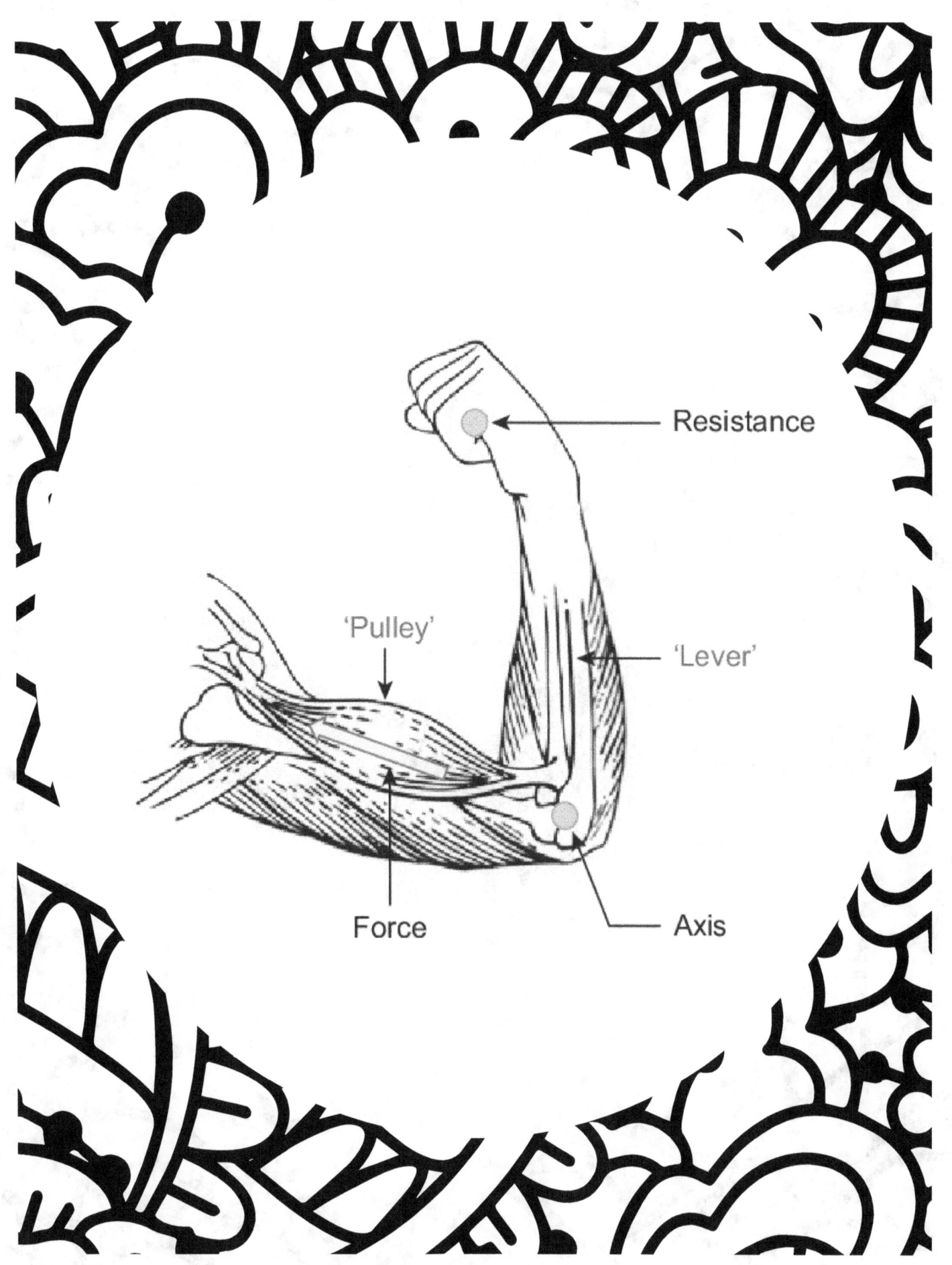

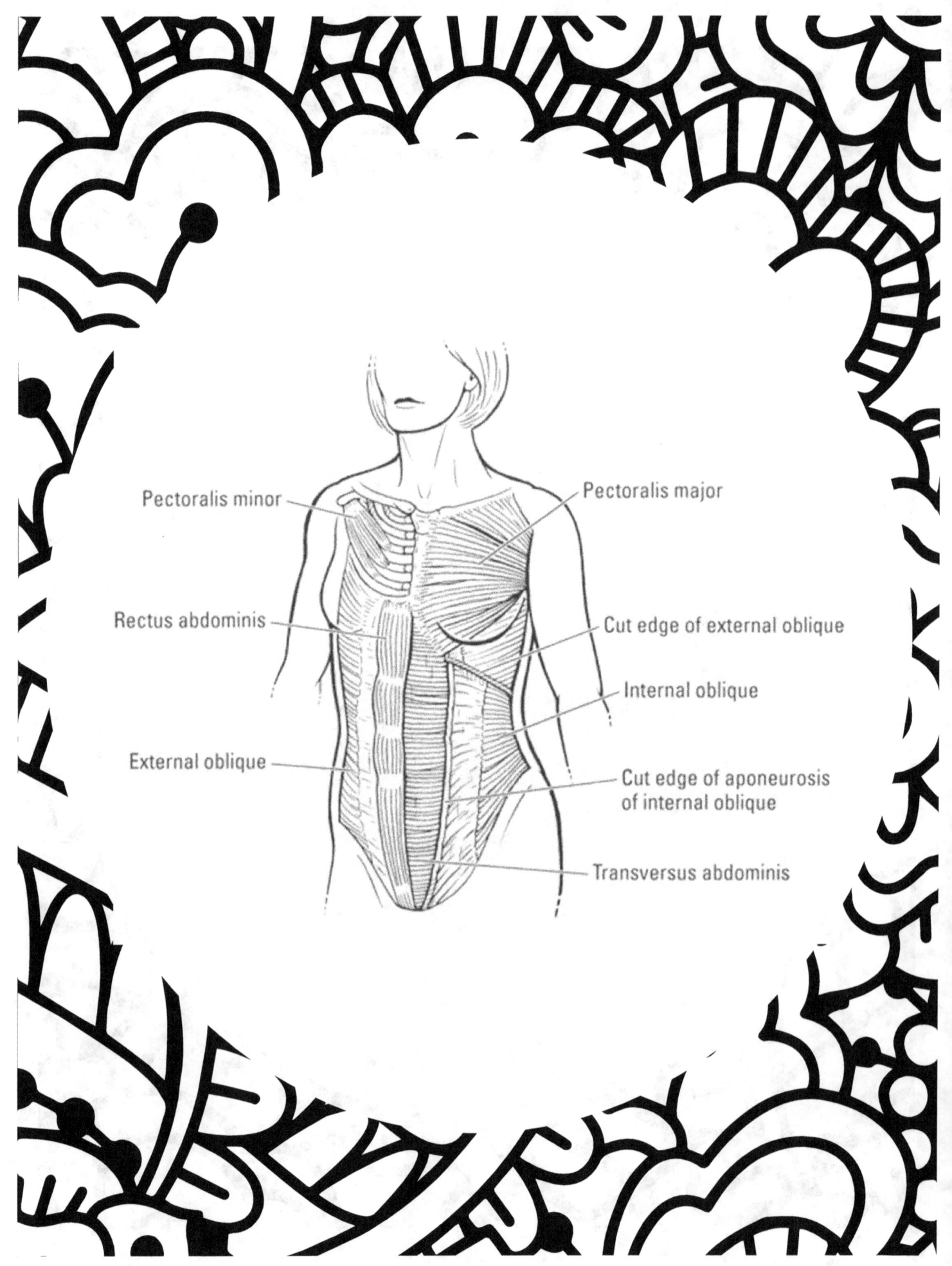

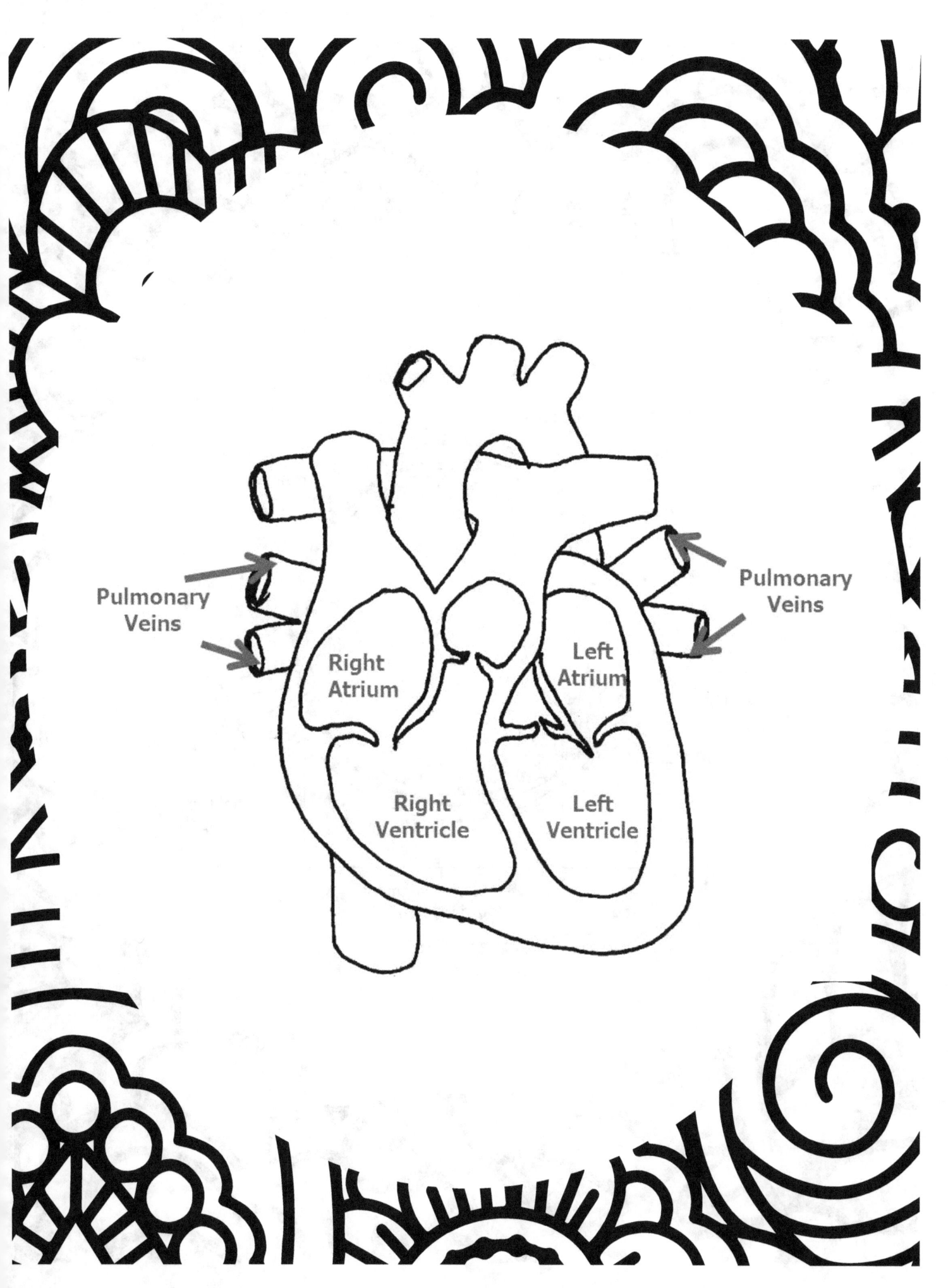

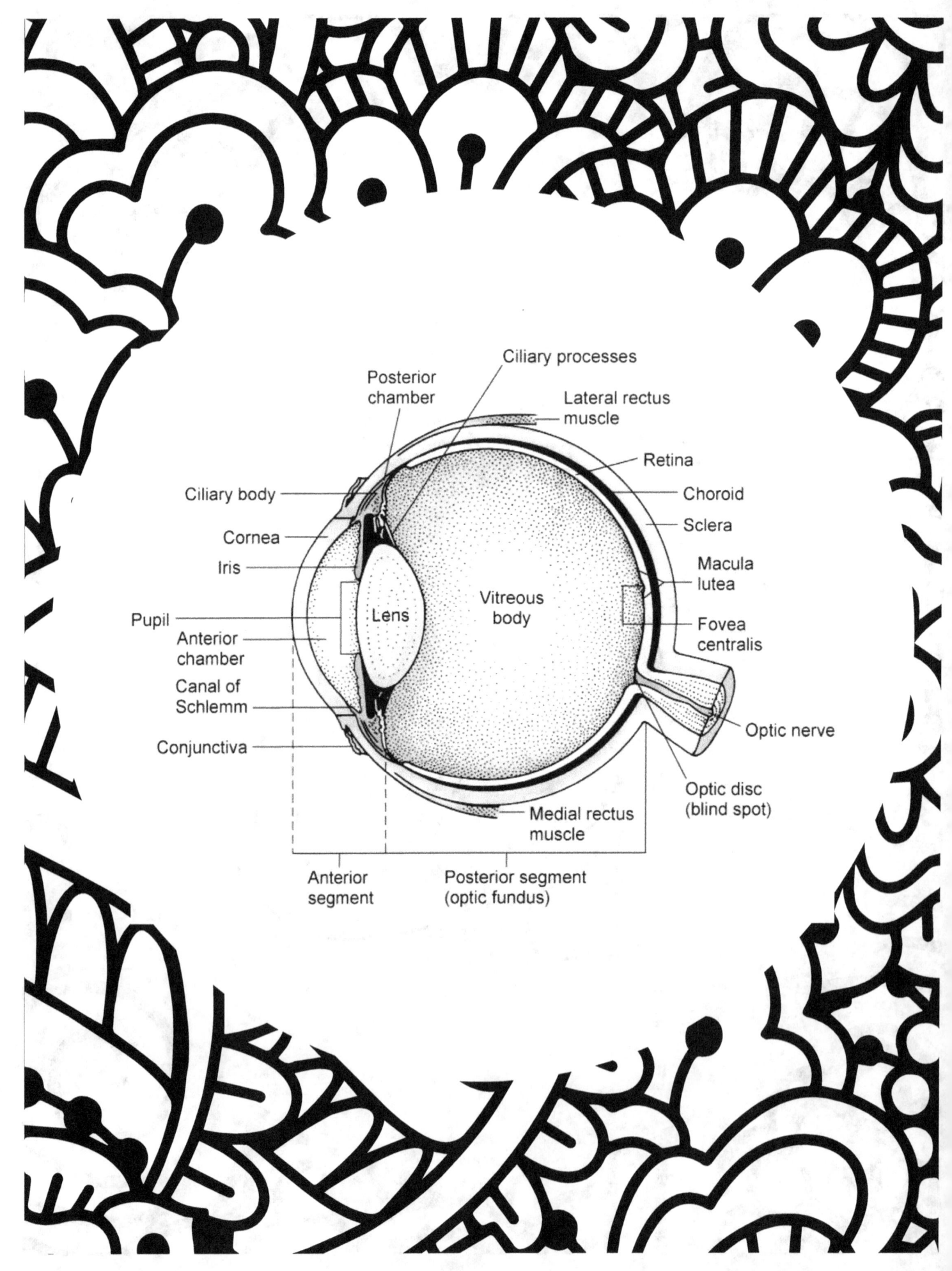

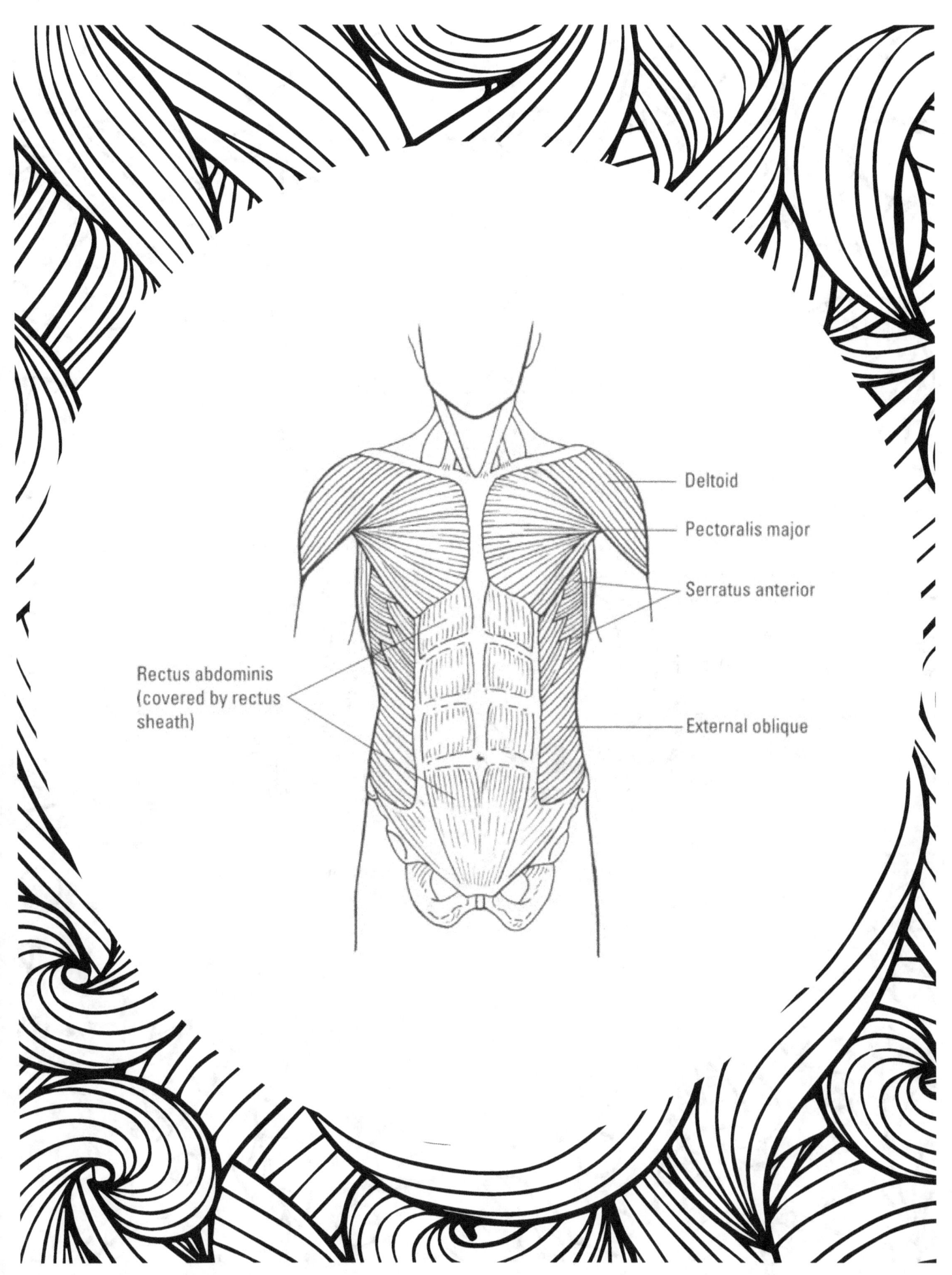

Deltoid

Pectoralis major

Serratus anterior

Rectus abdominis
(covered by rectus
sheath)

External oblique

Anatomy of the Human Eye

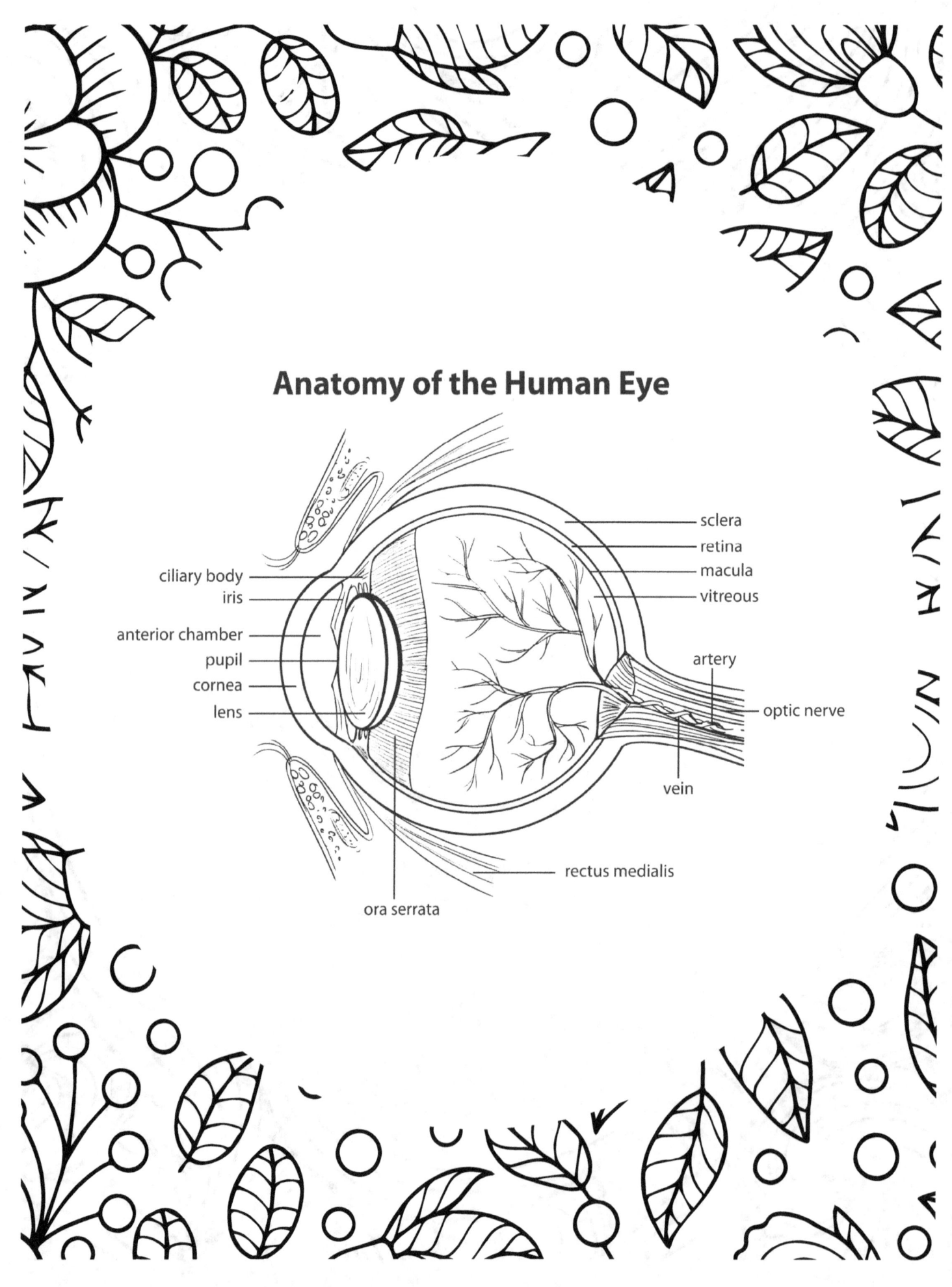

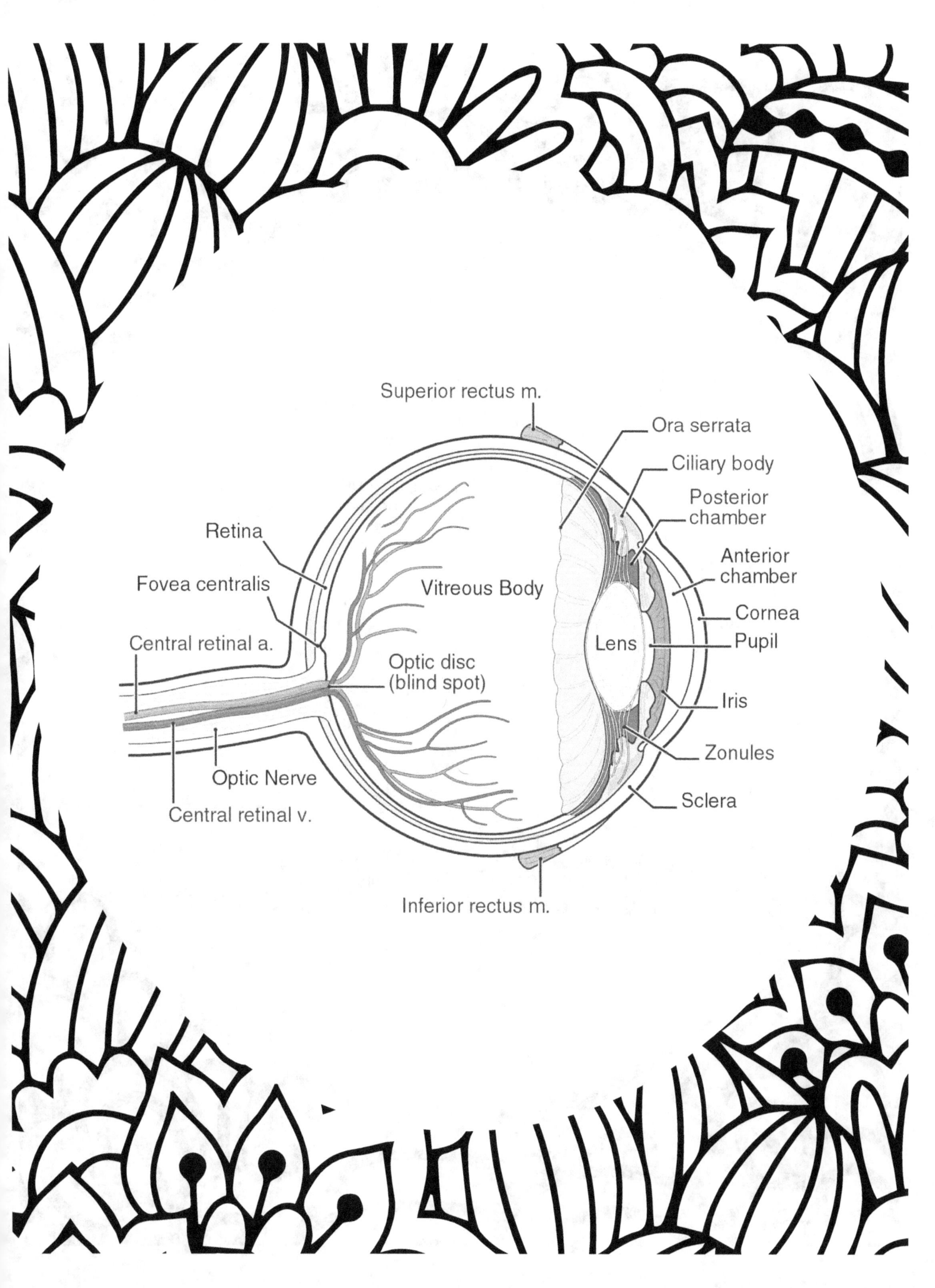

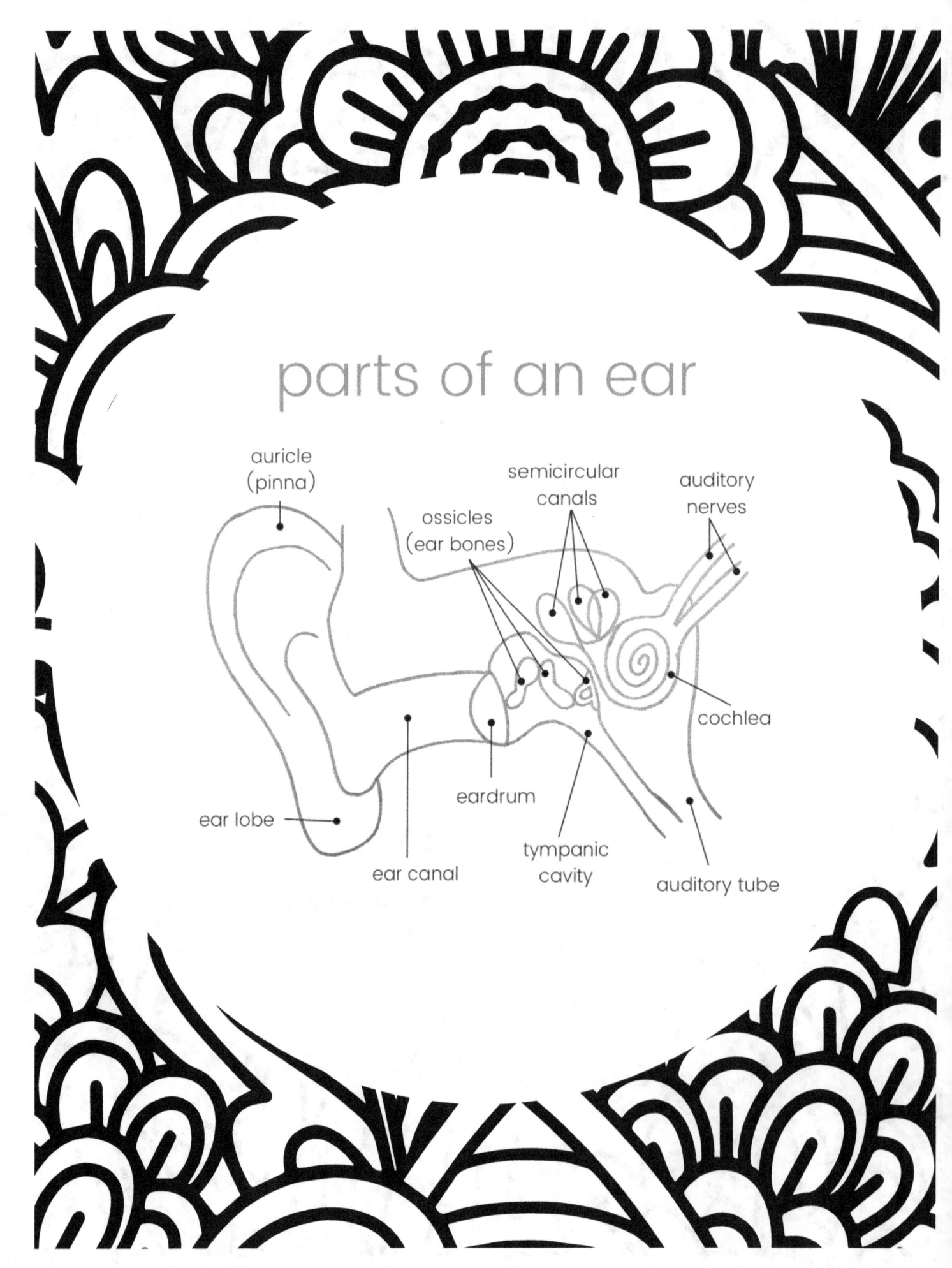

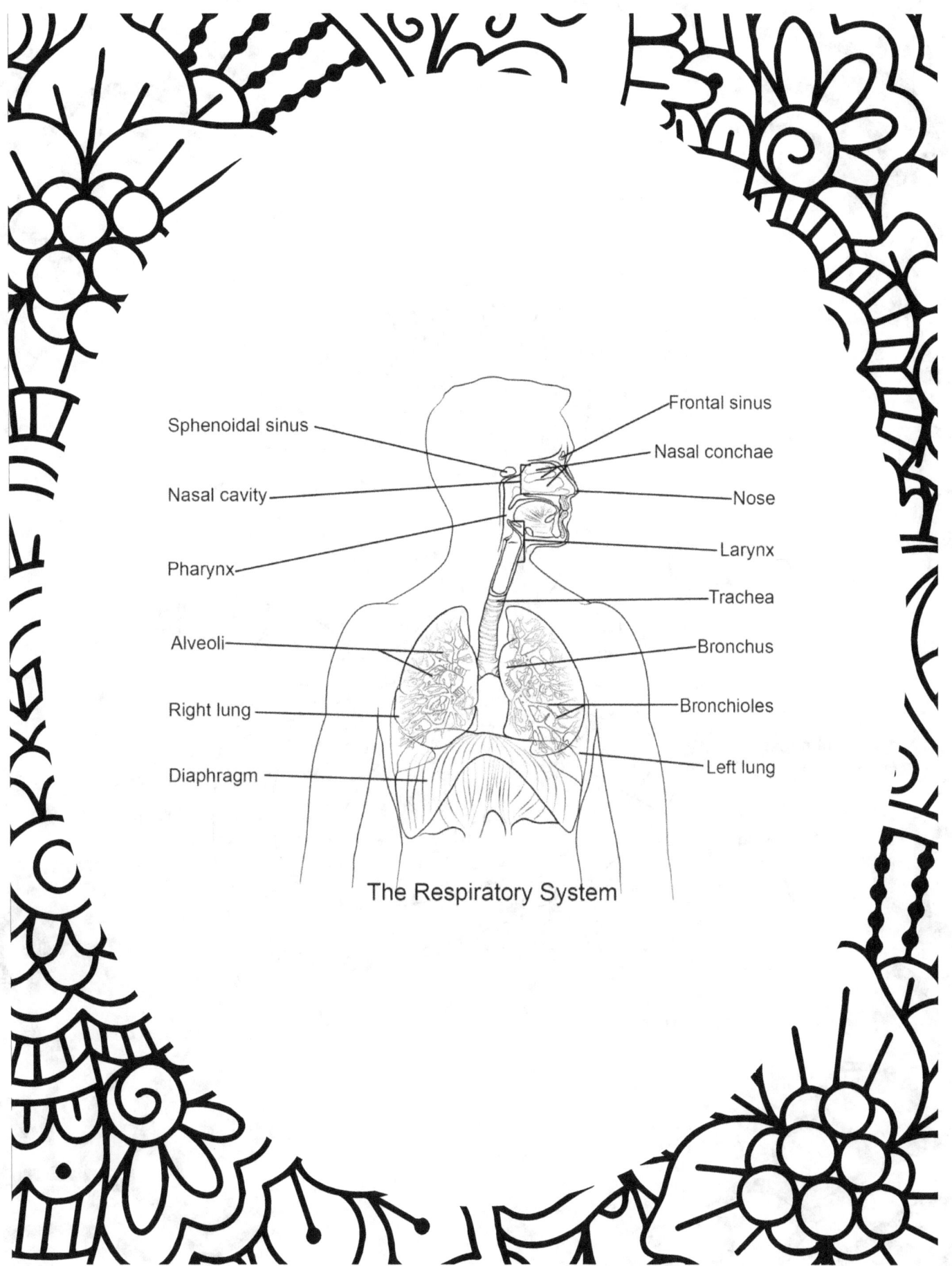

The Respiratory System

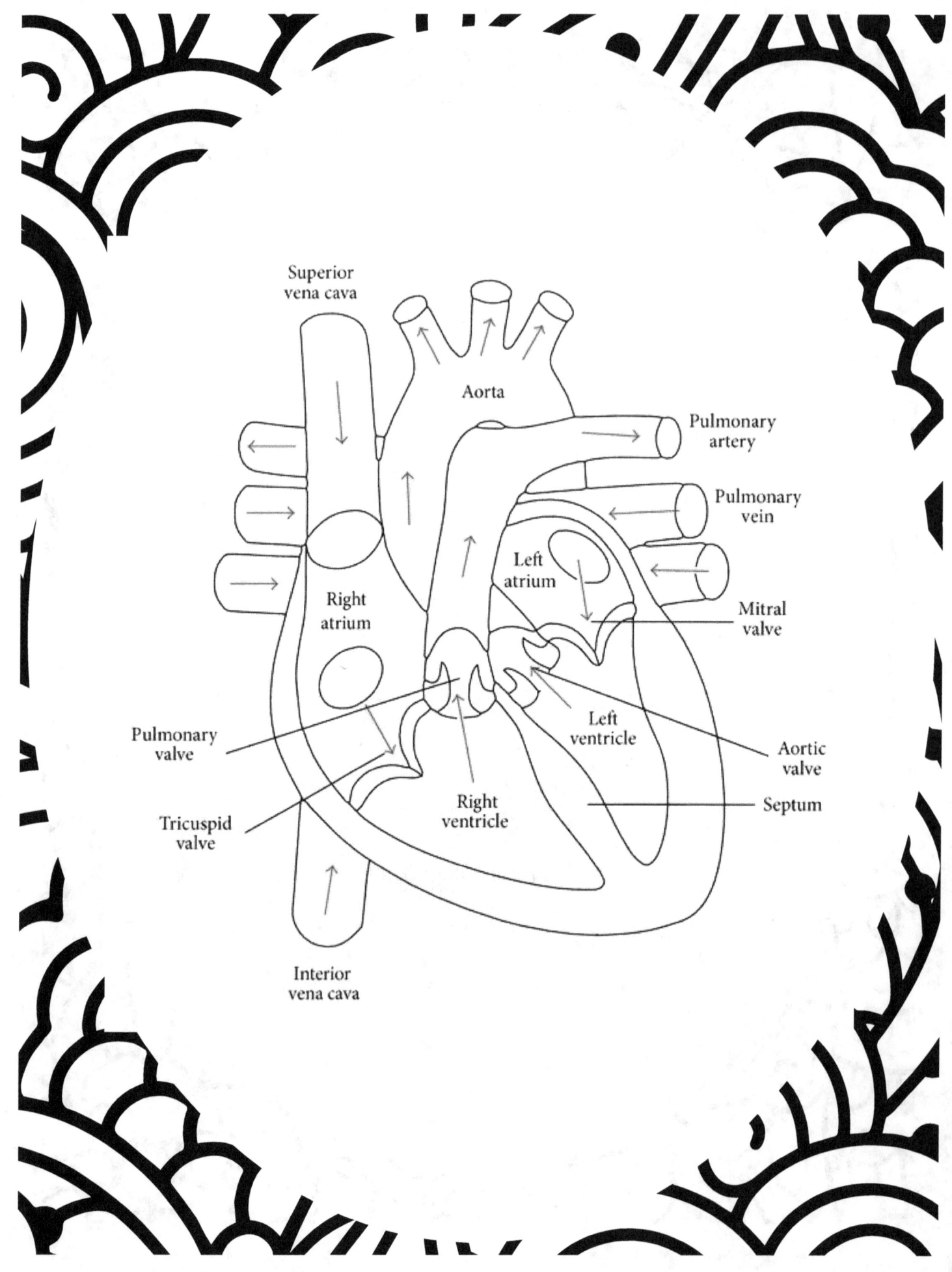

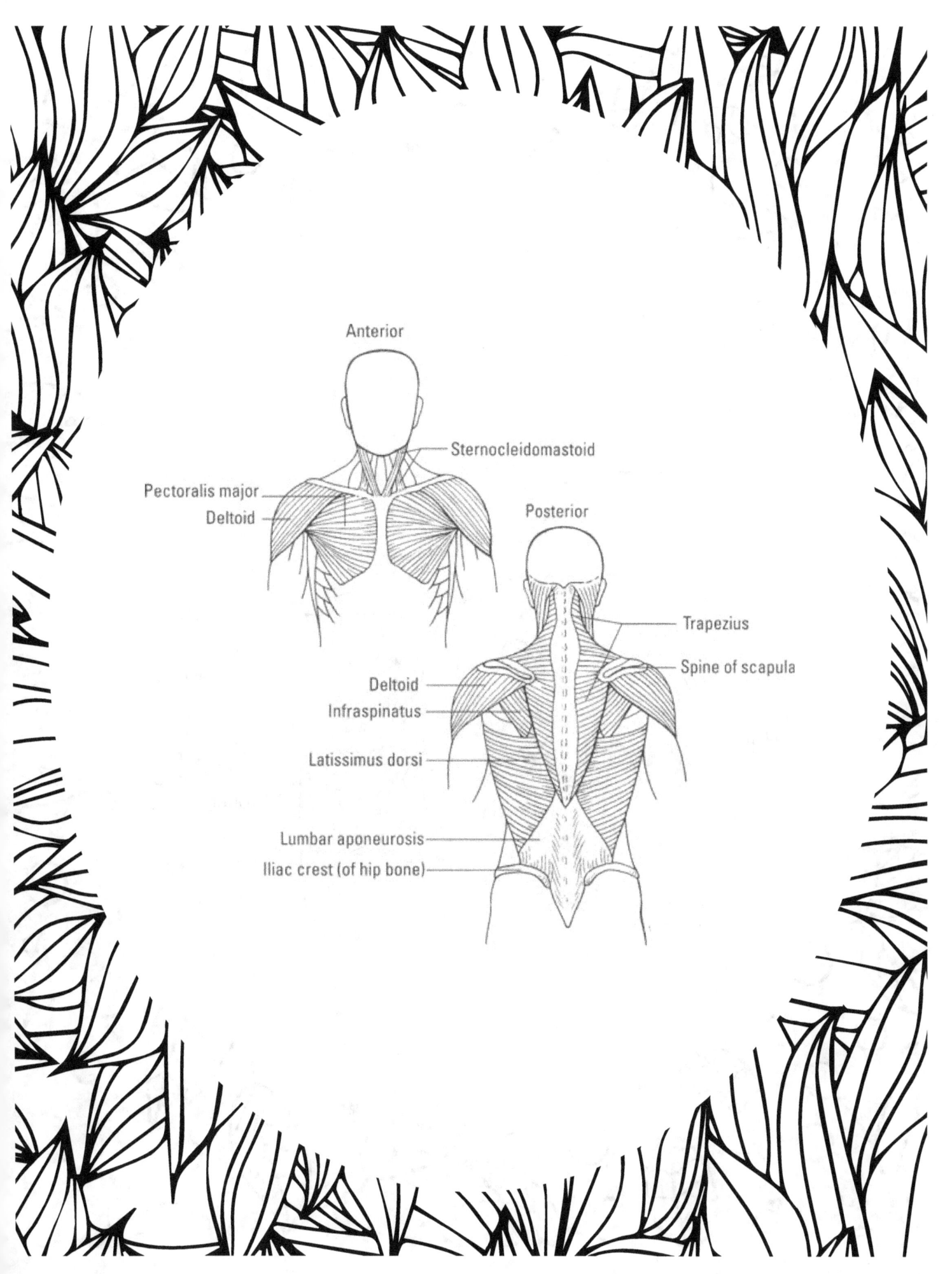

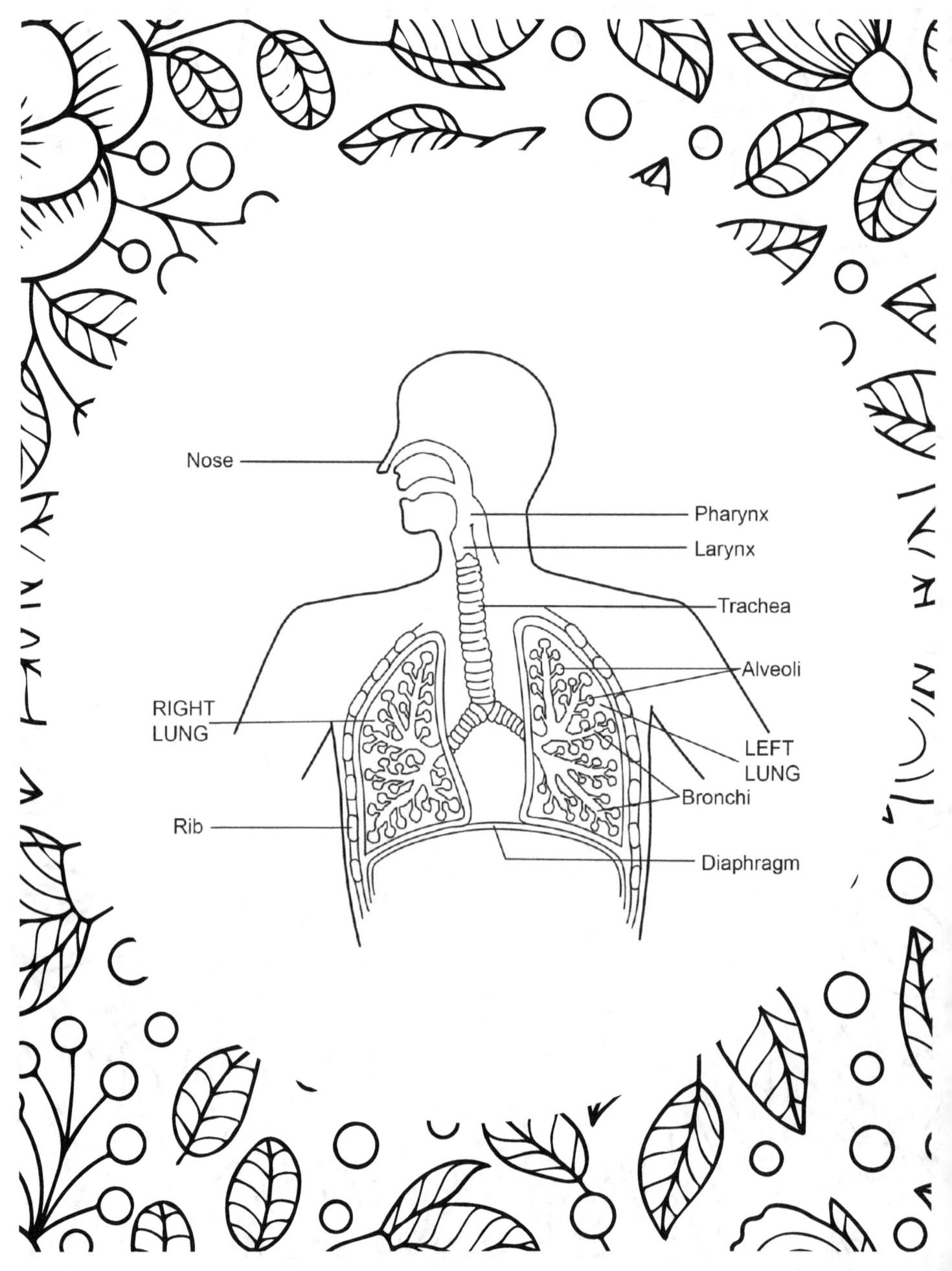

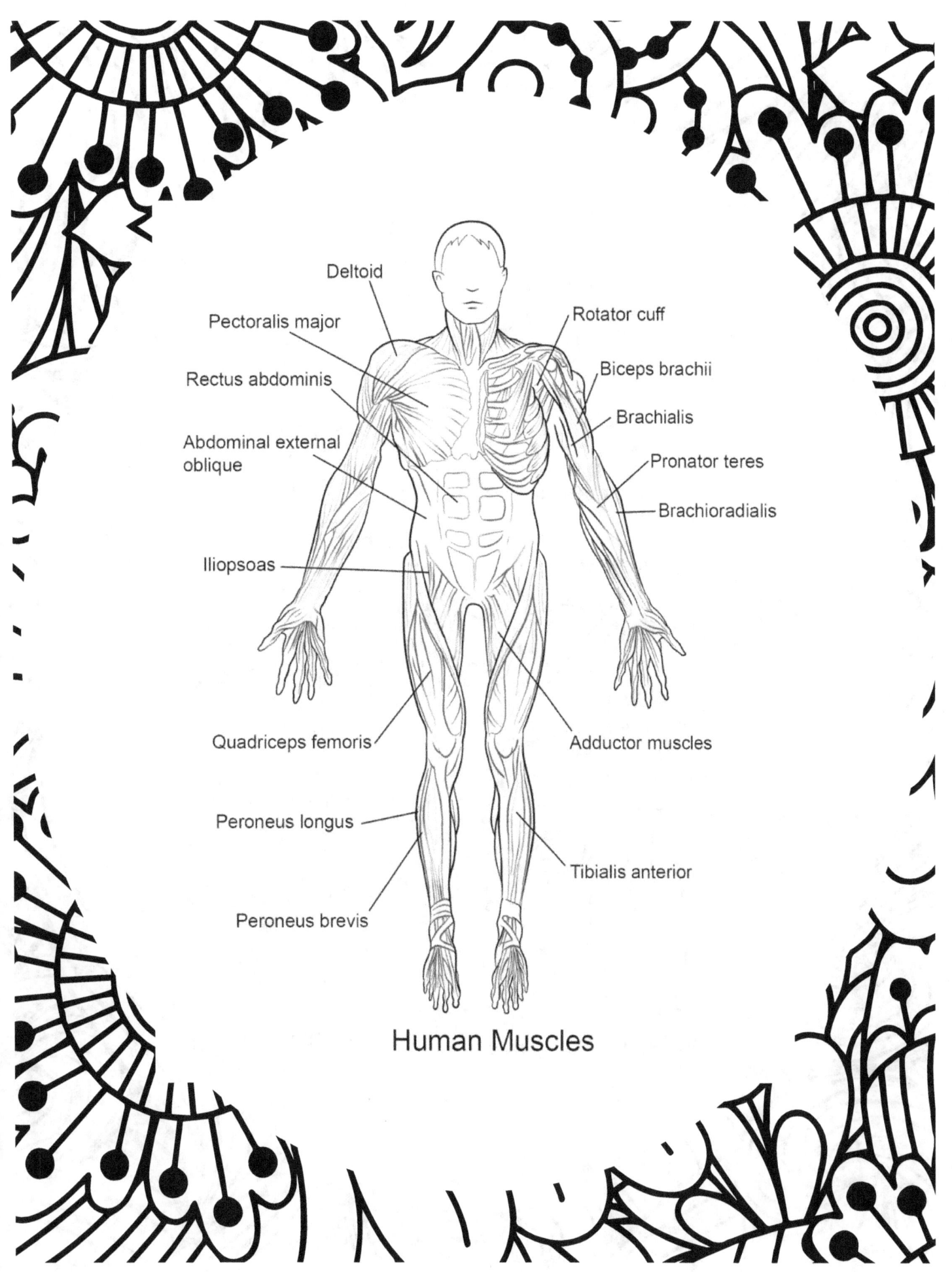

Human Muscles

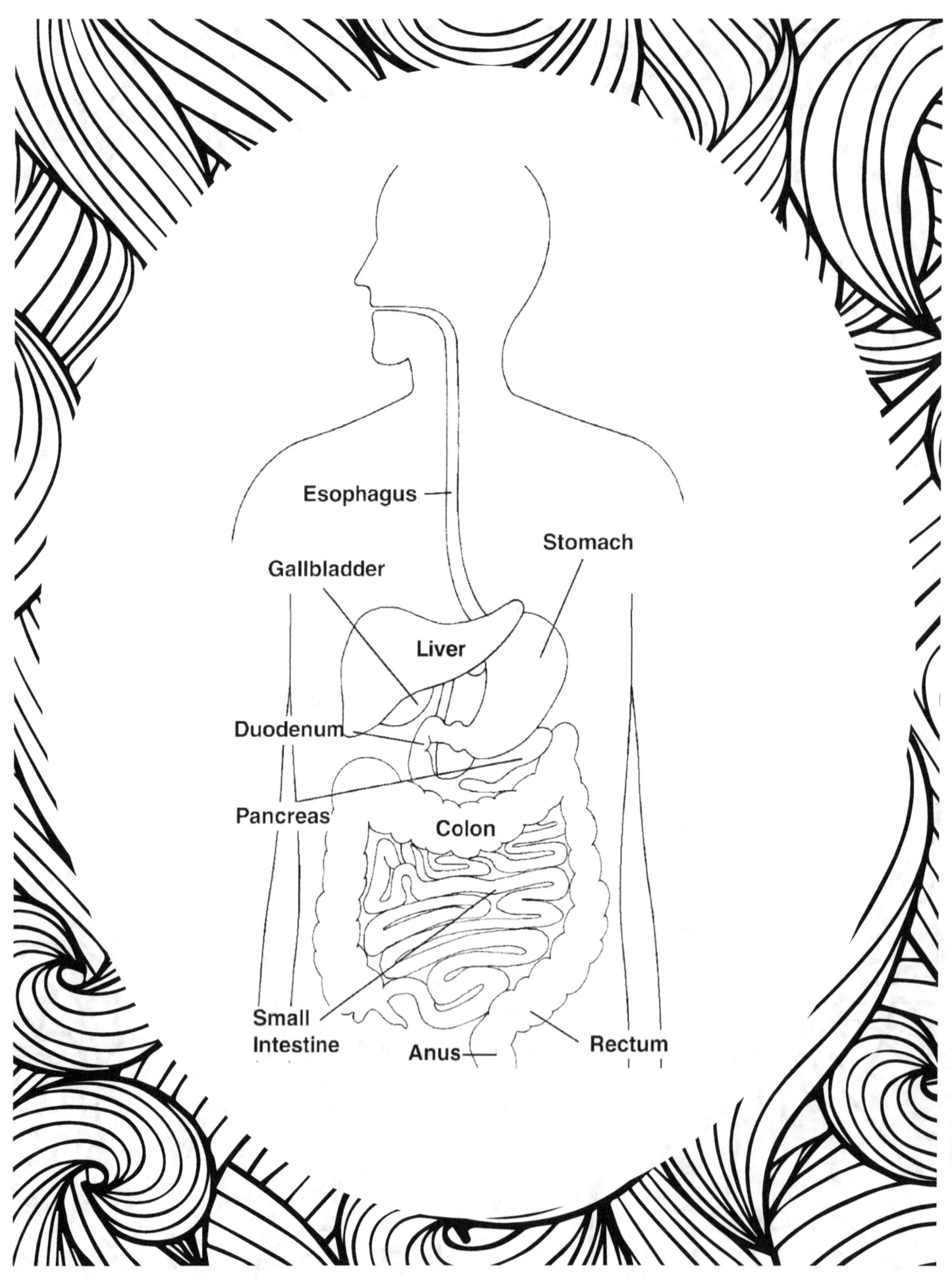

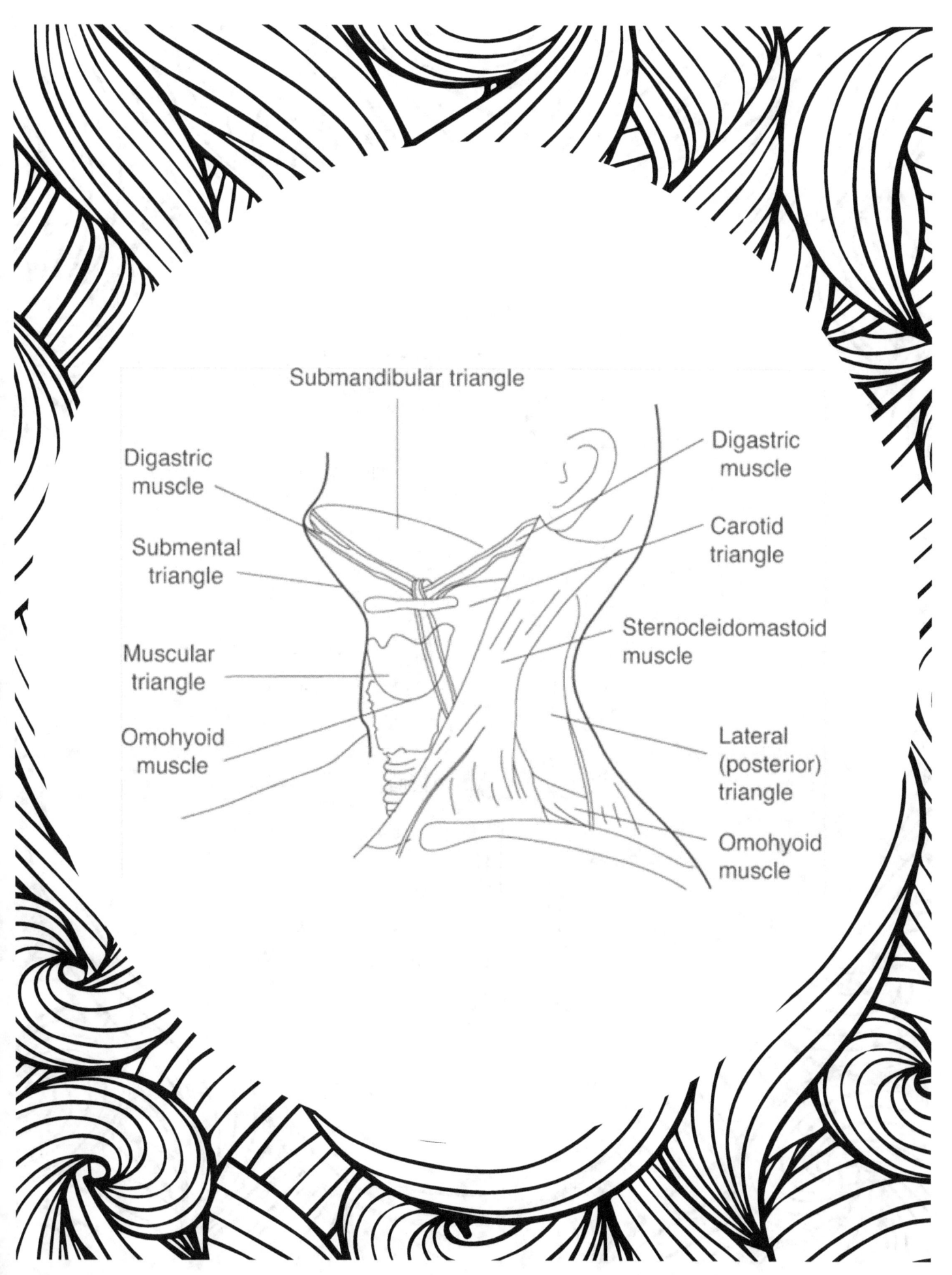

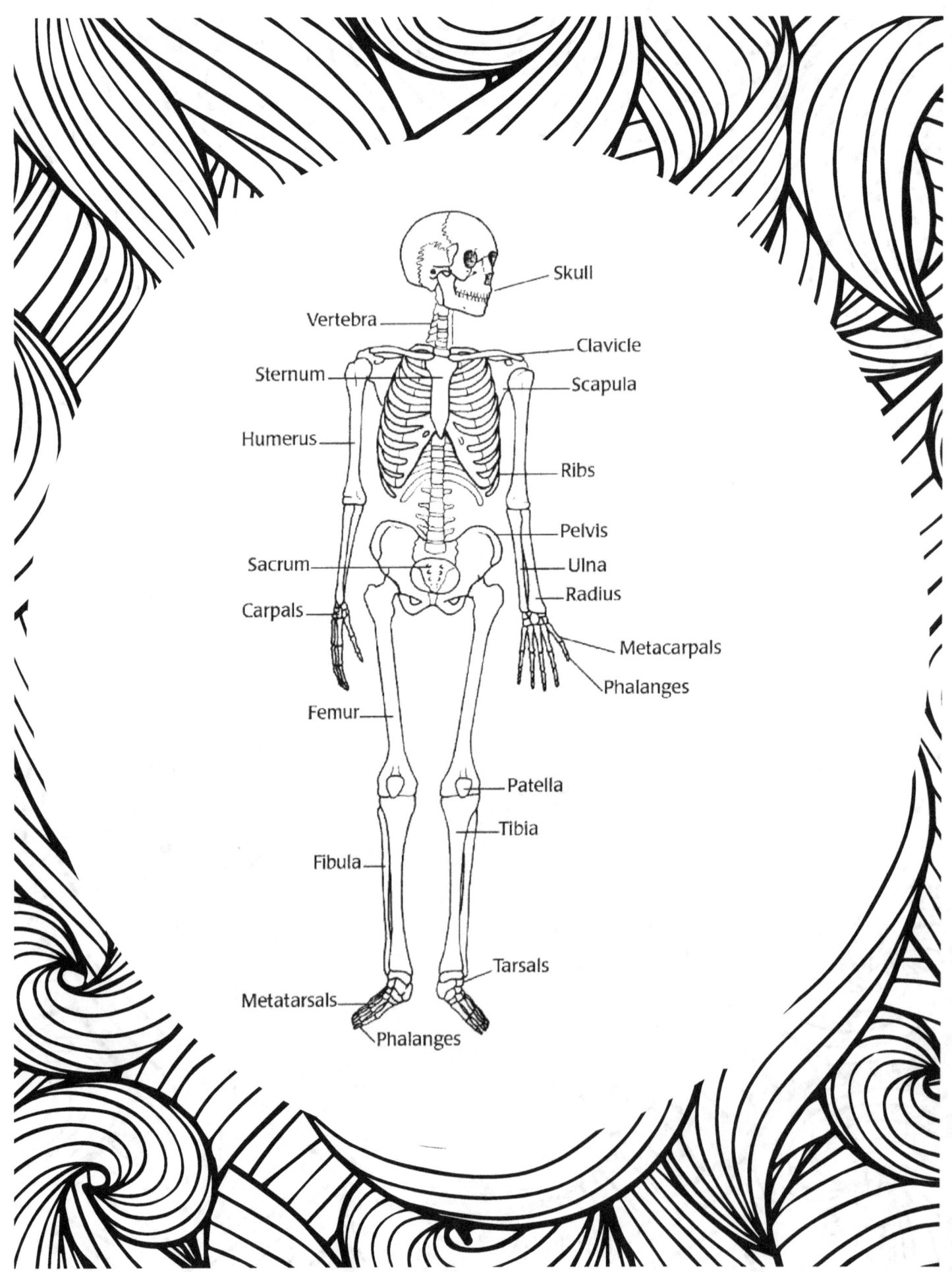

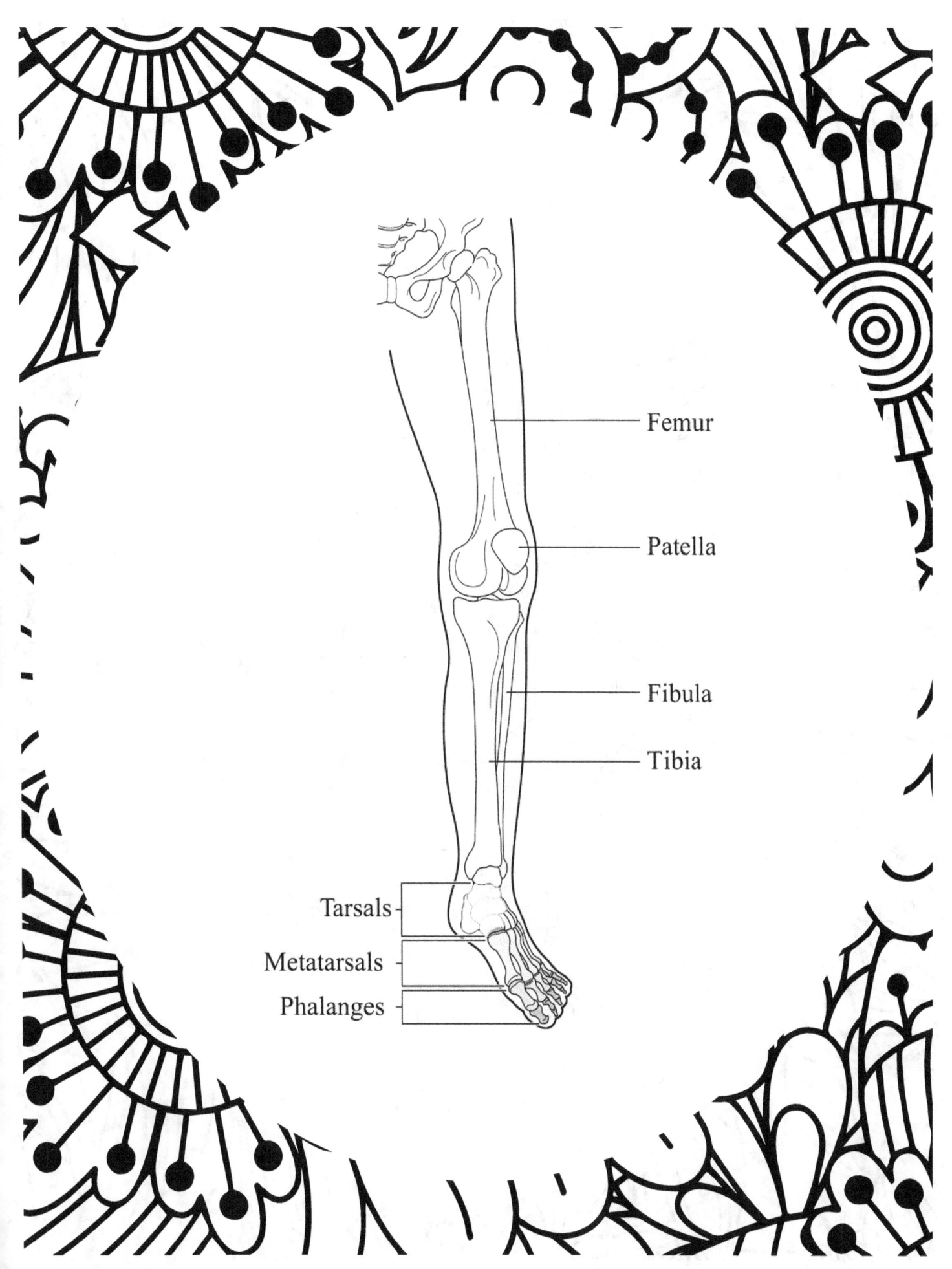

Femur

Patella

Fibula

Tibia

Tarsals

Metatarsals

Phalanges

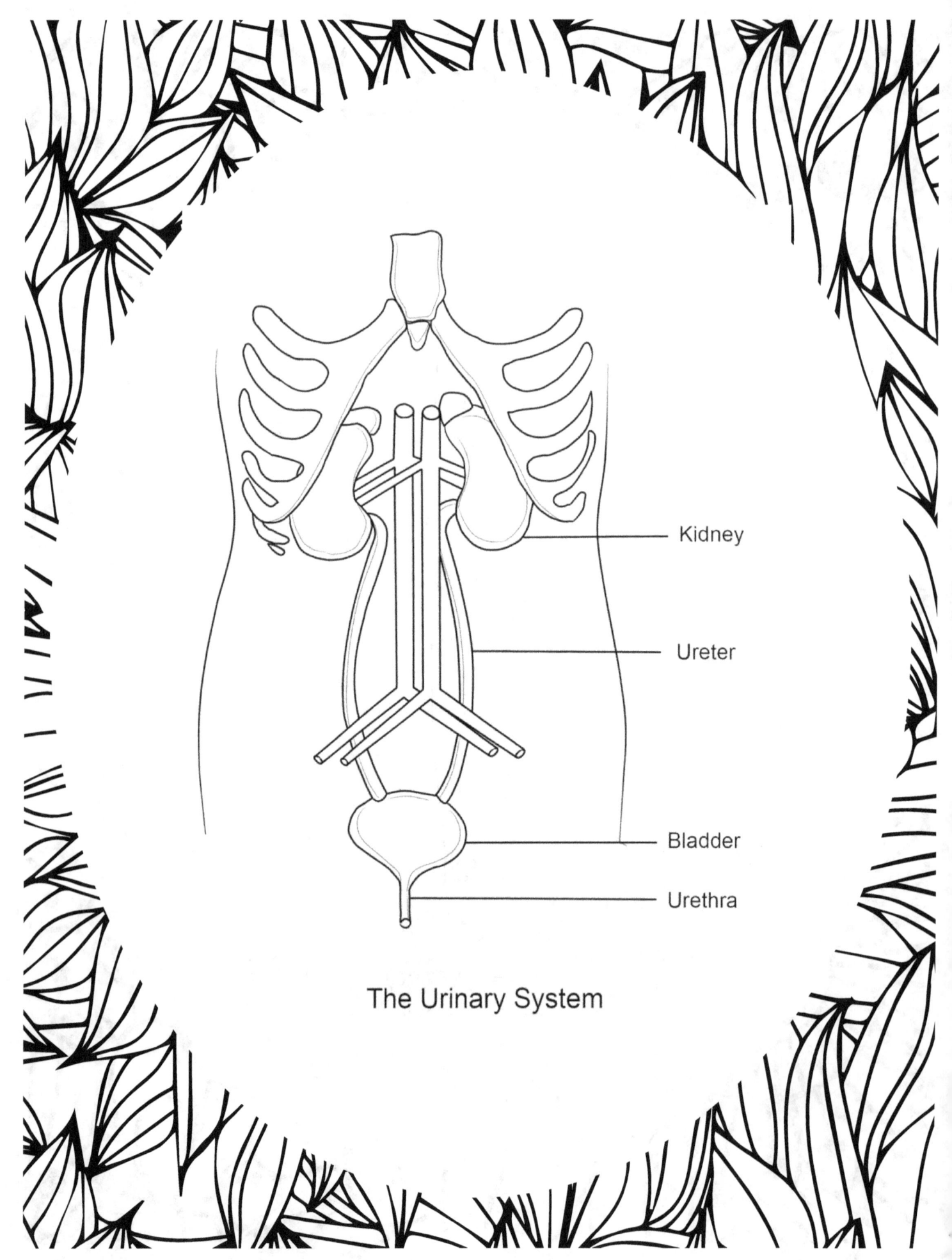

Kidney

Ureter

Bladder

Urethra

The Urinary System

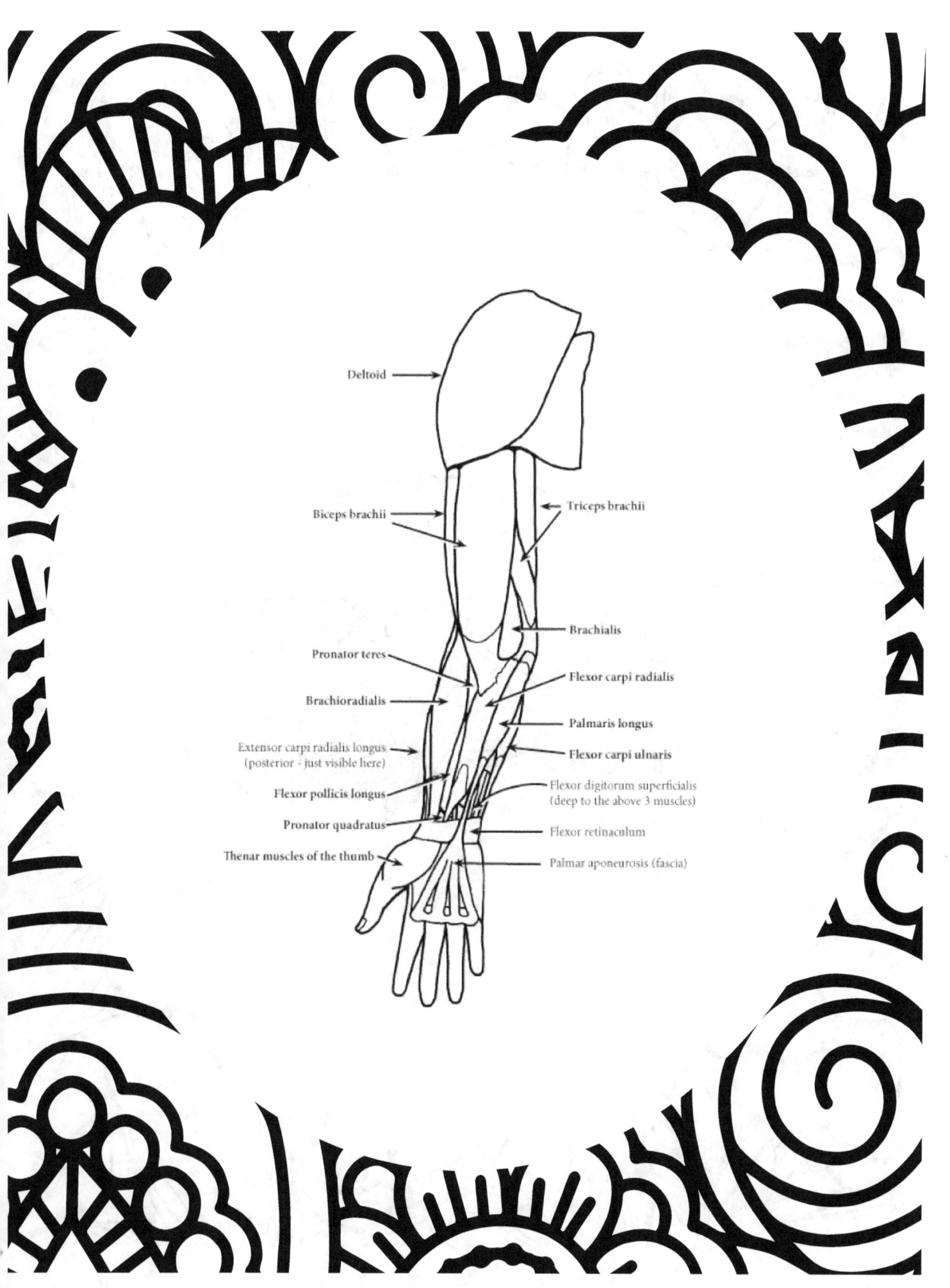

Deltoid

Biceps brachii

Triceps brachii

Brachialis

Pronator teres

Flexor carpi radialis

Brachioradialis

Palmaris longus

Extensor carpi radialis longus
(posterior - just visible here)

Flexor carpi ulnaris

Flexor pollicis longus

Flexor digitorum superficialis
(deep to the above 3 muscles)

Pronator quadratus

Flexor retinaculum

Thenar muscles of the thumb

Palmar aponeurosis (fascia)

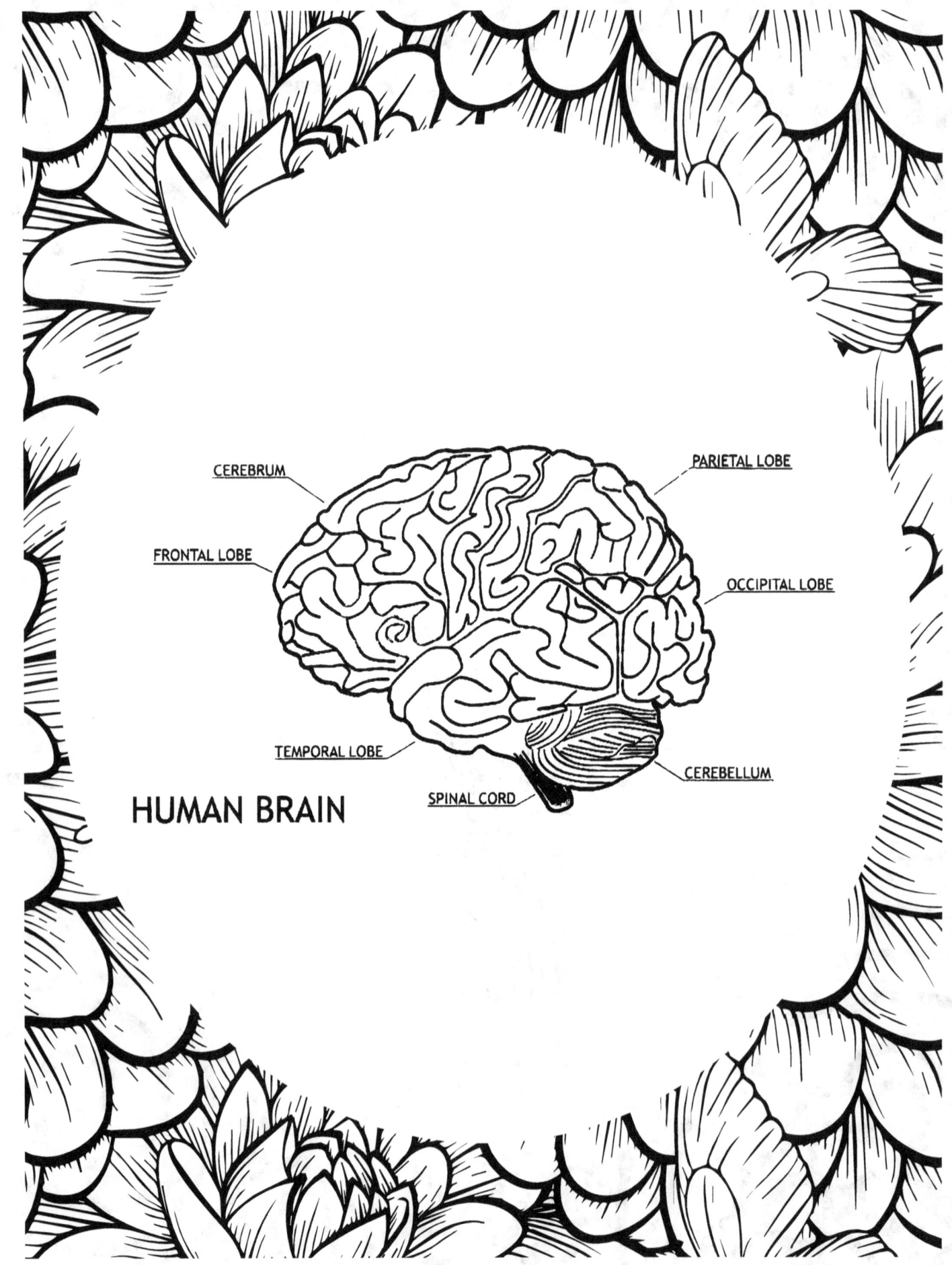

CEREBRUM

PARIETAL LOBE

FRONTAL LOBE

OCCIPITAL LOBE

TEMPORAL LOBE

CEREBELLUM

SPINAL CORD

HUMAN BRAIN

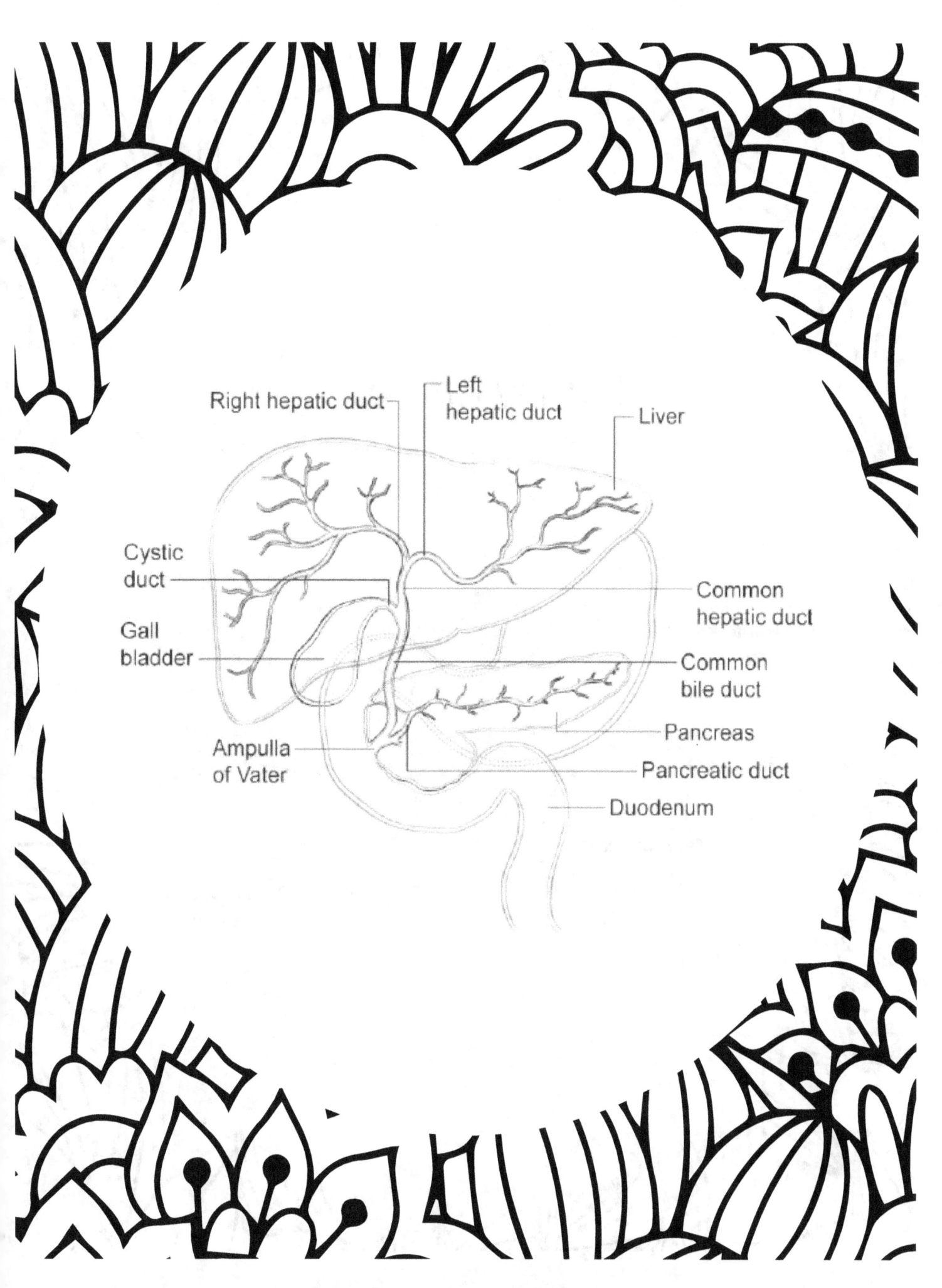

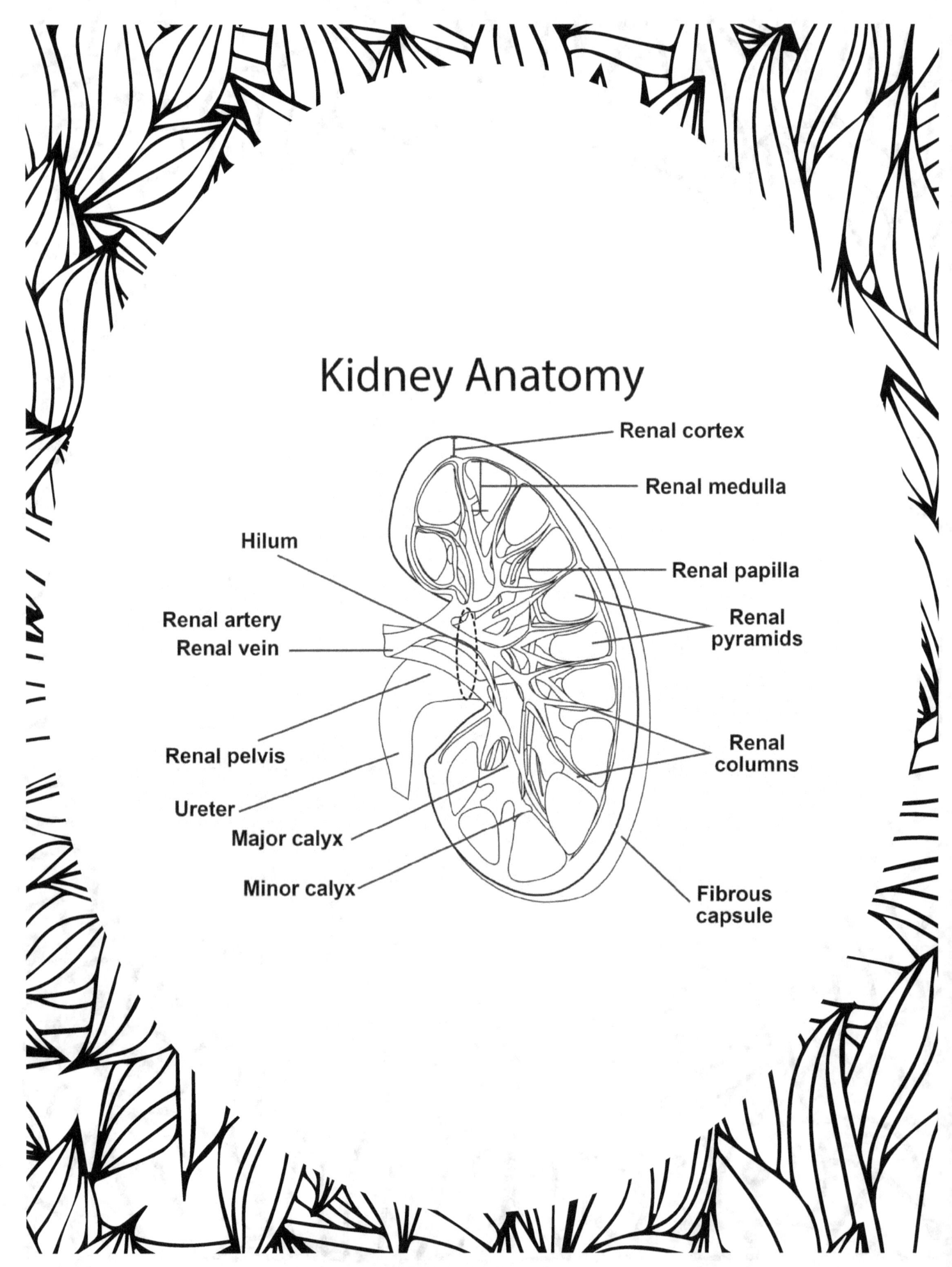

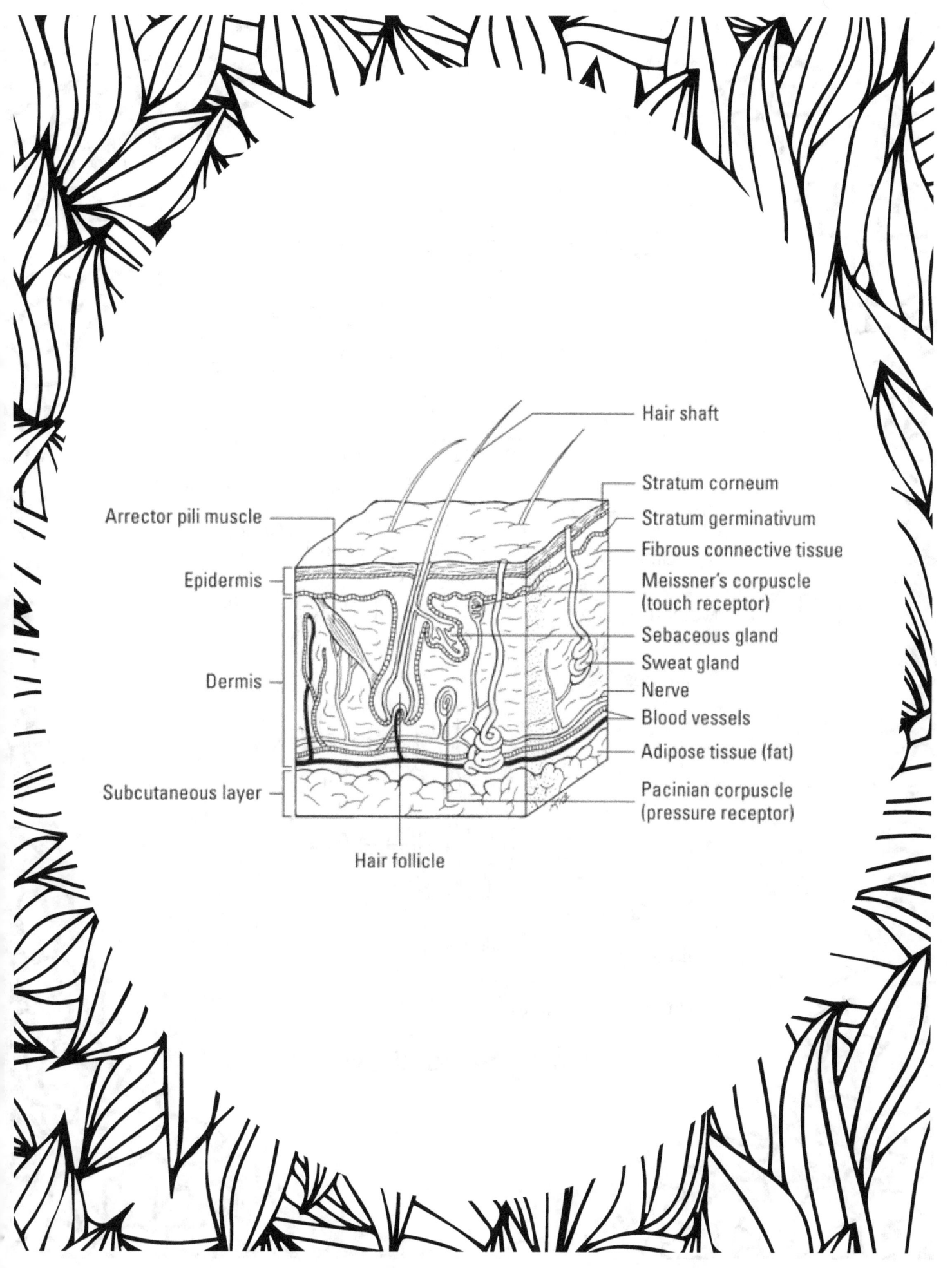

Hair shaft

Stratum corneum

Stratum germinativum

Fibrous connective tissue

Meissner's corpuscle (touch receptor)

Sebaceous gland

Sweat gland

Nerve

Blood vessels

Adipose tissue (fat)

Pacinian corpuscle (pressure receptor)

Arrector pili muscle

Epidermis

Dermis

Subcutaneous layer

Hair follicle

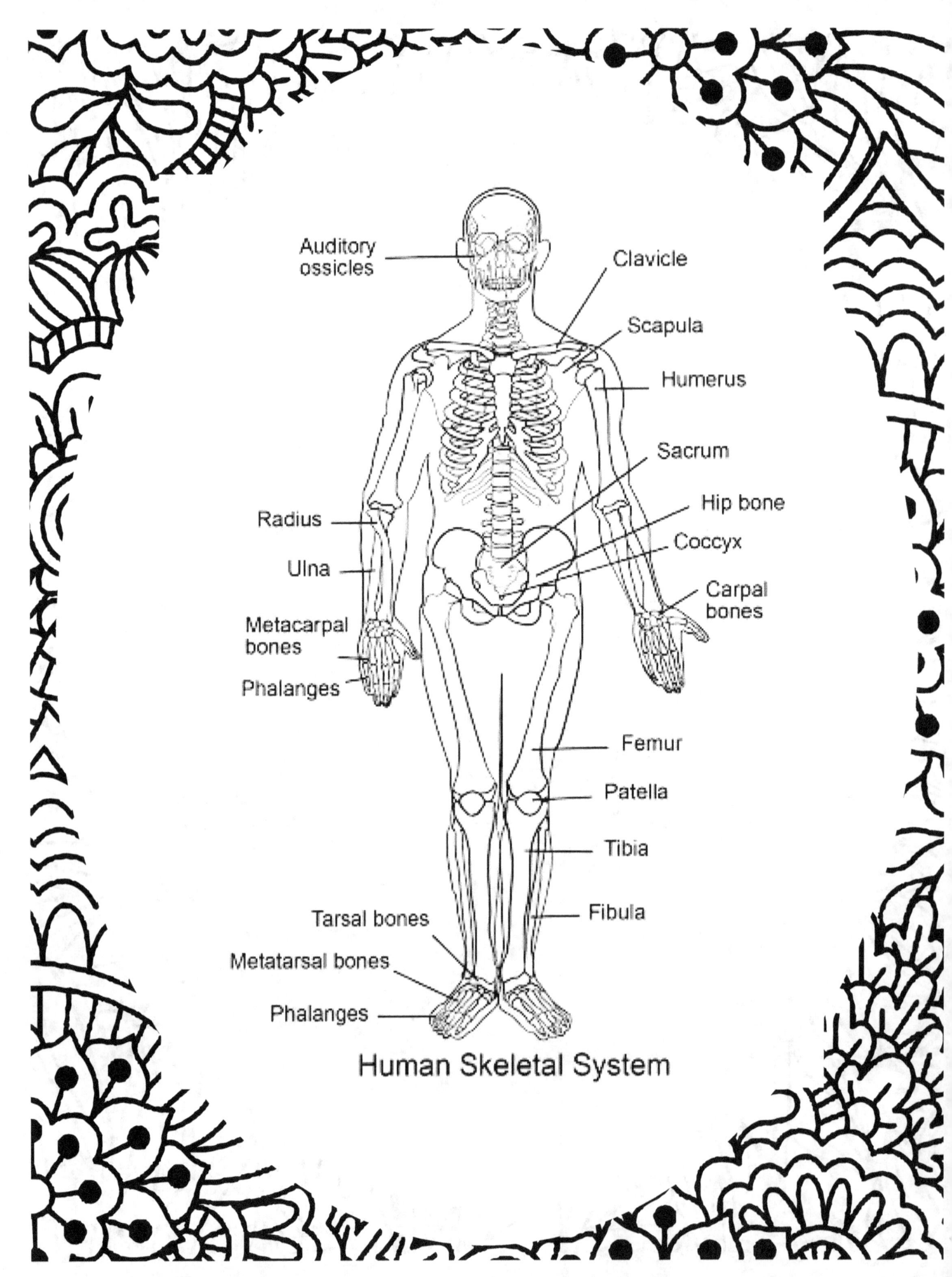

Human Skeletal System

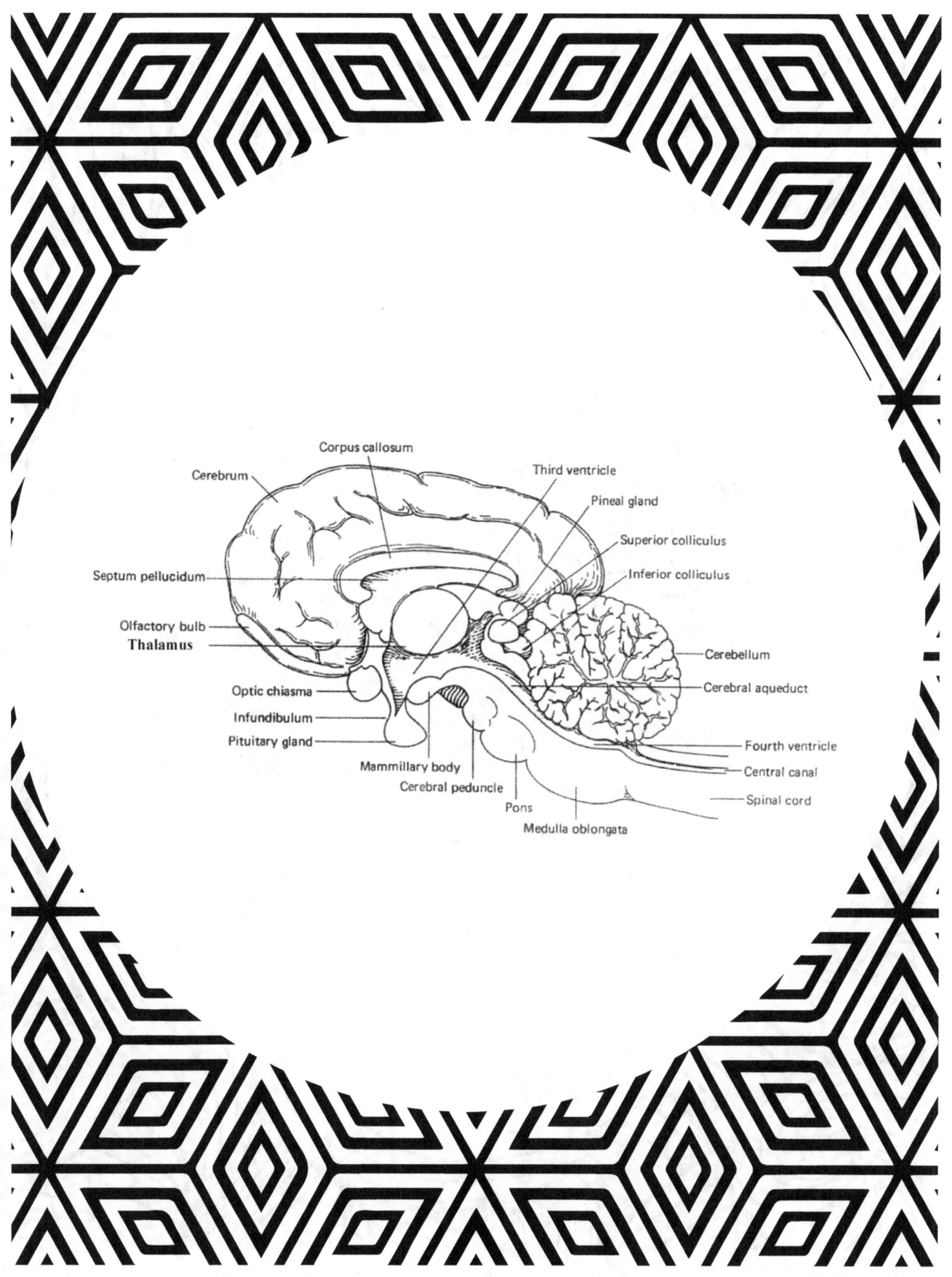

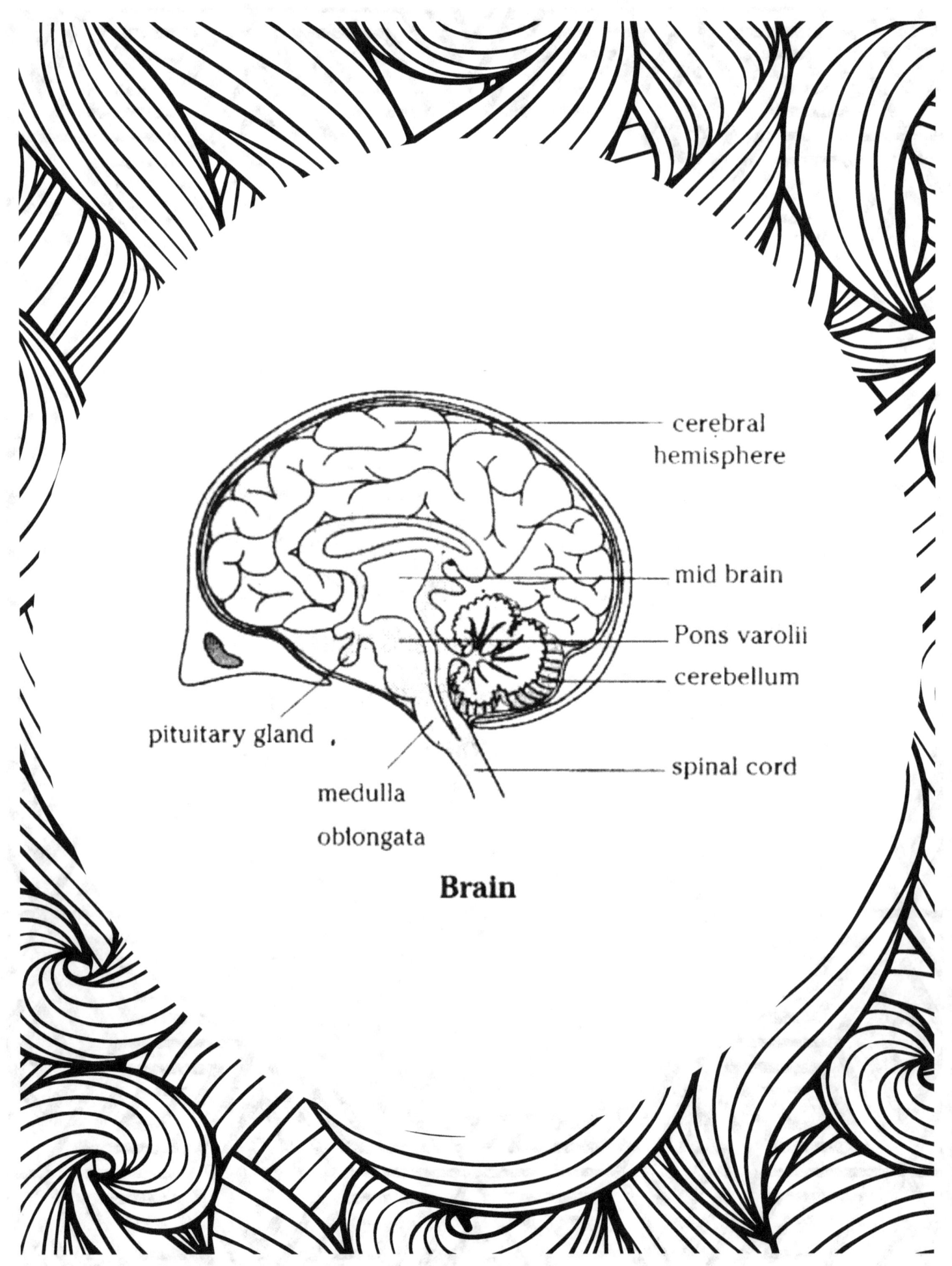

Brain

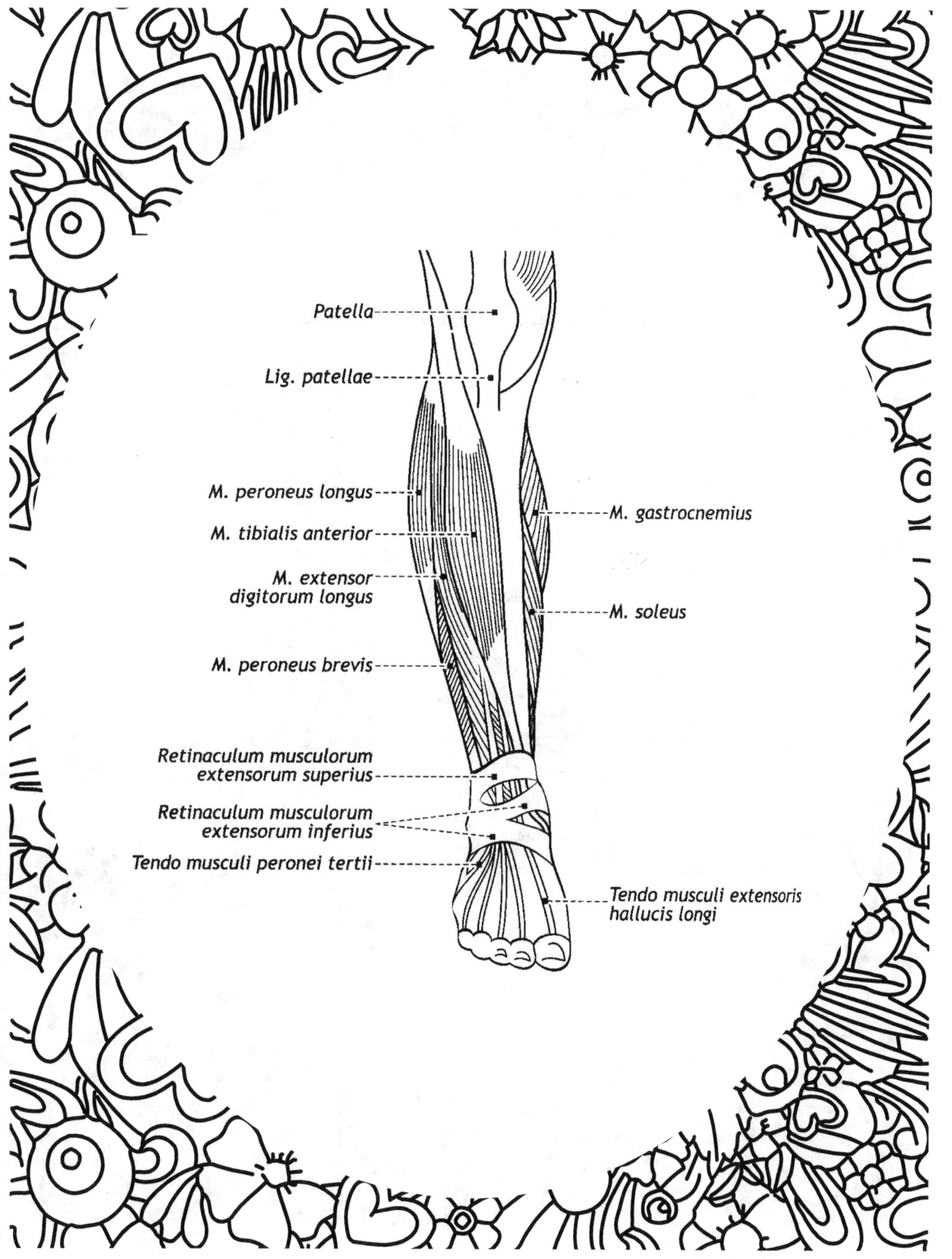

Patella

Lig. patellae

M. peroneus longus

M. tibialis anterior

M. extensor
digitorum longus

M. peroneus brevis

Retinaculum musculorum
extensorum superius

Retinaculum musculorum
extensorum inferius

Tendo musculi peronei tertii

M. gastrocnemius

M. soleus

Tendo musculi extensoris
hallucis longi

Color the Digestive Tract

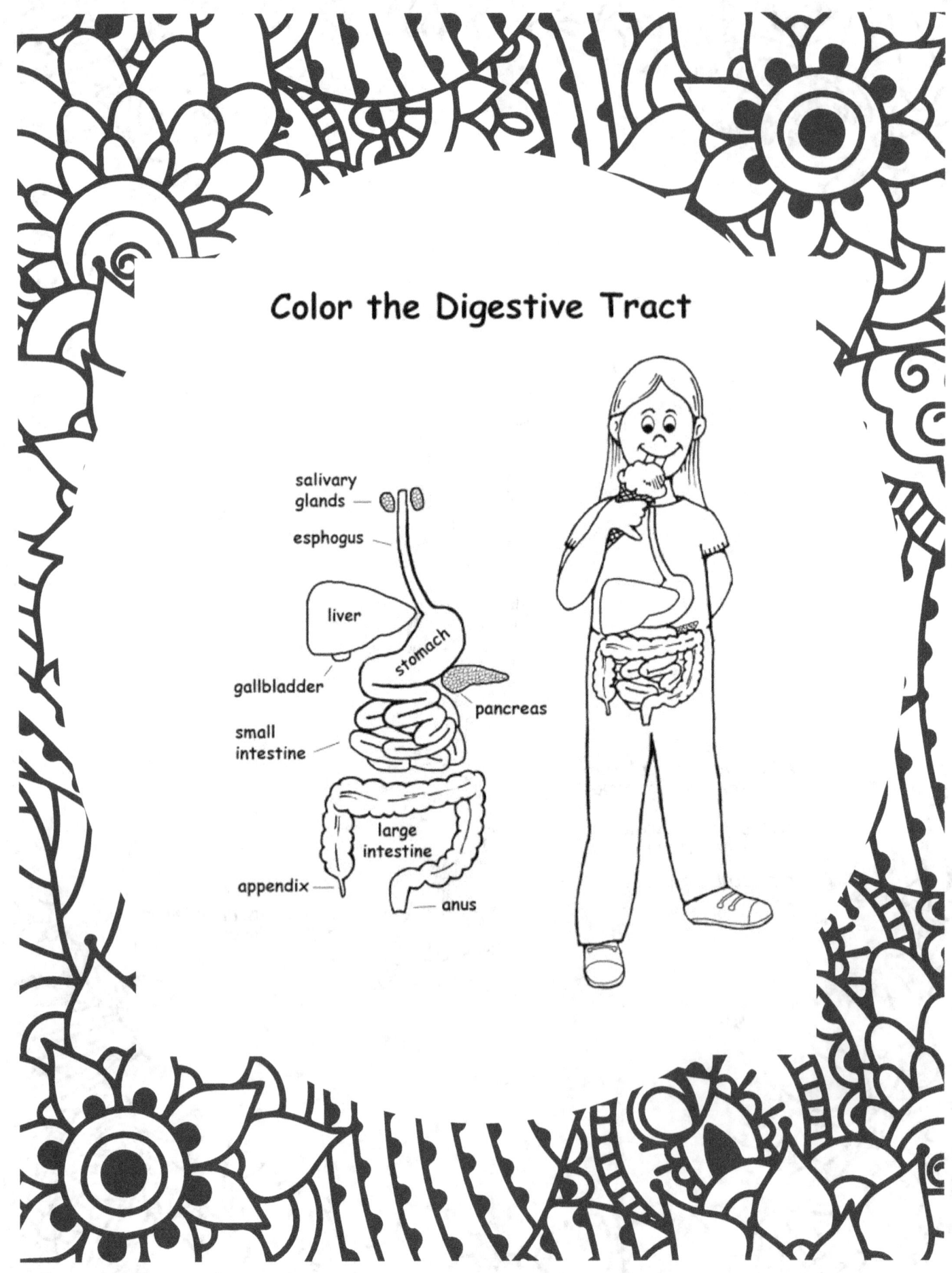

salivary glands

esphogus

liver

stomach

gallbladder

pancreas

small intestine

large intestine

appendix

anus

www.ingramcontent.com/pod-product-compliance
Lightning Source LLC
Chambersburg PA
CBHW081700220526
45466CB00009B/2838